The Healing Art
of
Writing

Perspectives in Medical Humanities

Perspectives in Medical Humanities publishes scholarship produced or reviewed under the auspices of the University of California Medical Humanities Consortium, a multi-campus collaborative of faculty, students and trainees in the humanities, medicine, and health sciences. Our series invites scholars from the humanities and health care professions to share narratives and analysis on health, healing, and the contexts of our beliefs and practices that impact biomedical inquiry.

General Editor

Brian Dolan, PhD, Professor of Social Medicine and Medical Humanities, University of California, San Francisco (UCSF)

Forthcoming Titles

The Remarkables: Endocrine Abnormalities in Art
By Carol Clark and Orlo Clark

Hatching Innovation: One Institution's Paths to Discovery
By Henry Bourne (Winter, 2012)

Clowns and Jokers Can Heal Us: Comedy and Medicine
By Albert Howard Carter III (Winter, 2012)

Social Medicine and the Politics of Health
By Dorothy Porter (Spring, 2012)

Darwin and the Emotions: Mind, Medicine and the Arts
Edited by Angelique Richardson and Brian Dolan (Fall, 2012)

www.medicalhumanities.ucsf.edu

brian.dolan@ucsf.edu

This series is made possible by the generous support of the Dean of the School of Medicine at UCSF, the Center for Humanities and Health Sciences at UCSF, and a MCRP grant from the University of California Office of the President.

The Healing Art
of
Writing

Edited by

Joan Baranow, PhD

Brian Dolan, PhD

David Watts, MD

Volume One

First published in 2011

by UC Medical Humanities Consortium and distributed by UC Press.

BERKELEY — LOS ANGELES — LONDON

© 2011

University of California

Medical Humanities Consortium

3333 California Street, Suite 485

San Francisco, CA 94143-0850

Cover Art by Anthony Russo, 2010

Library of Congress Control Number: 2011929102

ISBN 978-0-615-38132-9

Printed in USA

Contents

Brian Dolan

Preface

The Perspectives in Medical Humanities book series promotes scholarship produced or reviewed under the auspices of the University of California Medical Humanities Consortium (UCMHC)—a multi-campus organization that was established upon the principle of collaboration between scholars within the humanities and the biomedical and health sciences.

Our books investigate social, cultural and artistic meanings of health care and are primarily concerned to demonstrate how scholars from both the humanities and health-professions can speak to each other, and indeed a general audience, with minimal technical jargon and specialized academic language. Our series brings together the visions and analytic approaches from scholars across the "two cultures" divide to demonstrate how multiple perspectives enhance our overall understanding of certain themes or specific topics. Our commitment is not only to bridge disciplines, but to demonstrate how different perspectives complement and help inform each other. Thus we put into practice one of the central tenets of our pedagogical mission which is reflexivity: writing about how our own methods of understanding the topics we are researching change as the result of engaging with other points of view.

It is a great pleasure to introduce this, our first volume in the series. *The Healing Art of Writing* brings together caregivers and patients who share a passion for writing about the mysterious forces of illness and recovery. A belief shared among all contributors is that being cured of a disease is not the same as being healed, and that writing poetry and prose brings us to a place of healing. Our writers embrace perfectly what our series aims to promote, which is the desire to communicate to audiences beyond any individual academic or professional community in order to share perspectives on the cultures of health and healing that profoundly impact so many lives.

The editors would like to thank the University of California Office of the President's Multi-campus Research Program Initiative for funding the UC Medical Humanities Consortium that supports this series. We would like to thank Laura Cerruti, Director of Digital Content Development, at UC Press, as well as Matthew Winfield, Operations Coordinator at California Digital Library, for their support.

Joan Baranow and David Watts

Introduction

In the summer of 2010 a group of writers, poets, patients, nurses, and physicians gathered for a week-long conference on the campus of Dominican University of California to explore through writing the various dimensions of illness and healing. They were drawn together by a shared belief that expressive writing has the power to heal the spirit. Many also believed that writing is an act of courage and that facing one's illness is the first step towards healing the body. Poets were encouraged to write new poems daily and to share their poems in a workshop setting. Prose writers brought manuscripts for detailed discussion. Some of the participants were seasoned writers and poets; others were sharing their writing for the first time. It was a week of exploration and discovery, revelation and support.

The Healing Art of Writing celebrates the writing that emerged during that week. Among the nearly one hundred contributions you will find poems that speak of suffering, loss, and compassion; memoirs that describe childhood pain, nights in the ER, sudden illness, and caring for loved ones. You will also find faculty lectures that tie our personal stories to the larger world of literary expression. These are stories of survival and joy, offered in the spirit of healing.

David Watts

The Healing Art of Writing

My journey into writing was precipitous and unexpected. I'd been suffering a few flesh wounds from a mid-life crisis and couldn't understand why it was having such an effect on me. Somehow, and without understanding why, I had a feeling that writing might help clear up a few things. So I started to make a few poems.

Basically, they sucked, which I thought was unfortunate, and which probably damaged my ego a little, and dashed my hopes for something artistic and lasting. But all that didn't seem to matter, because I continued deriving benefit from the process even so, feeling less pressured or less discombobulated even while making some pretty horrible scribbles on the page. When I started looking at these snippets from a critical perspective it was clear I didn't know what I was doing. So I did the logical next thing: I went out and got some craft.

Things started getting better.

Over time I migrated from poetry to NPR commentaries, to non-fiction short stories to memoir and eventually a novel, never having planned *any* of that. It was clear I was hooked and loving my brand new tattoo. The personal benefit from writing, like a sustained absinthe rush, continued right along. That was impressive enough by itself but what struck me was that I didn't have to be producing Pulitzer Prize material to derive personal profit.

So how does *that* work?

My son, in his bed at night, three years old, always asked for "a growing up story." Usually he made his request when he had had some tough experience during the day, someone was mean, some difficult idea like war or death crossed his path, or maybe it was just the occasional injustice of pre-school playgrounds ... somehow instinctively he knew there was something to be found there, some steadfast quality in these stories that would lull, or reassure, or heal.

Instinctive? So it would seem, this time early in the life of the next generation. So I wondered, what do my son's experience and mine have in common?

After 911 the sales of poetry books soared. That says to me that somewhere in our collective consciousness we know something about poems and stories ... deep down we know that they provide sustenance in times of crisis. Frost says that we don't look to poetry for solutions but for a pathway through. Whatever it is we look for, even that which we may not be able to put a finger on, we seem, nonetheless, to know where to find it.

It has something to do with language, I think, and the payload that language carries.

Evolution created this business of language. Suddenly we have a hand with a prehensile thumb so we need a tool. The tool needs a name. Then we need to distinguish one tool from another and among tools in general, farming tools from hunting tools from weapons of war, and so we begin to create abstractions to represent them and then we can decide to classify them. Once we have linguistic distinctions for objects—abstractions that take the place of the thing itself—we have the ability to make abstract concepts, to form a mental image of that object then develop conversations around complex systems of classification, analysis, and association ... which leads, ultimately, to a more amazing kind of abstraction, a concept of self.

As humans, we are aware of our environment, ourselves and our inner world. To be self-aware like that, and to know that we are self-aware ... that is consciousness.

Living things have *cognition* but not necessarily *consciousness*: the sunflower knows how to face the sun all day, the amoeba to withdraw from something sharp or toxic in the environment, but only the animal capable of language has consciousness. Consciousness is not a place but a concept. Not a location but a synthesis of diverse neural pathways. Not a thing but a process. It is inaccessible to neurophysiological analysis, chemistry or physics; it is accessible only to language.

And so we weave linguistic networks. We exist in language which in turn feeds into our consciousness. What we bring forth has to do not only with what we understand about our environment, but what we understand about our inner workings. We communicate information but at a more sophisticated level, a coordination of behaviors, or what is known as structural coupling.

The more we play with language the more it leads us further into abstract ideas. Which, it seems, judging from some of our behaviors in the world around us, may be both good and bad. We have intelligence, creativity, innovation, technology, cruelty, war, and suffering. We are the only species who systematically destroys other members of our own kind yet we build rocket ships and create beauty in the form of art. We can achieve reflection which allows us to assemble meaning out of things, to define a pattern of relationships.

So with consciousness we have this new level of knowledge, linguistic, which is sometimes in harmony and sometimes in conflict with our inborn, instinctive knowledge. There is a price to pay for this consciousness. We make inhibitions. We set up societies that have rules. We have restrictions. If we steal a pumpkin from the grocer it might make perfect sense in terms of survival, but it works against the goals of society. Lusting after your neighbor's spouse might make exquisite Darwinian logic, but is not permitted. We inhibit ourselves for the benefit of social harmony. Even language itself gets inhibited. "You know, Zeke, you just can't go around talking about that good-for-nothing grandson of yours that way. And for god's sake, don't you go getting politically incorrect on me."

Inhibitions, it turns out, are not healthy. Confrontations are. Confrontations force a rethinking of the events.

Some societies already know this. The Pre-Columbian Native Americans had complicated confession rituals. So, too, a number of world religions. Unburdening tensions through speaking the unspeakable produces a sense of relief, a release from tension, a shift toward contentment. Polygraph tests that generate confessions often produce a great sense of relief in their subjects, even gratitude for making life less complex.

A suggestion we might derive from all this is that if we confront our demons we will fair better. If that is so, language provides us the avenue. Breuer's famous "talking cure" demonstrates this idea.

Dr. Breuer's celebrated case was a woman who refused to drink water from a glass. Under hypnosis he induced her to talk about water, about glasses, and anything else she could think of related to that. During "talk-therapy" she recalled observing her dog lapping and slurping water from her dinner glass. Once she remembered this disgusting event and made the obvious mental connection, she no longer suffered from her phobia.

Freud's fascination with Breuer's case led him to develop psychotherapy in which talking leads to emotional connections which leads to insight which leads, when working at its best, to cure. Or at least, to better understanding.

Here are some modern examples. People who are able to talk about the loss of a spouse fair better than those who refuse to.[1] Employees caught in downsizing who talk about their anger, frustration, sense of betrayal, get rehired at a rate of 27% as opposed to 5% in those who do not.[2] Talking into a recorder about heavy issues is a cure for insomnia.

The psychologist James Pennebaker had asthma. He developed his attacks living in West Texas and attributed them to the dust that blew in from New Mexico. When he visited home during Christmas he could expect to get an attack, and usually did. It all made sense. But when his parents came to visit him in Florida, lo and behold,

---

1   James W. Pennebaker, *Opening Up: The Healing Power of Expressing Emotions*, (New York: Guilford Press, 1990), 23.

2   S. P. Spera, E. D. Buhrfeind, and J. W. Pennebaker, "Expressive writing and coping with job loss," *Academy of Management Journal*, 37 (1994): 722–733.

he got an asthma attack. It wasn't the dust from New Mexico. It was his parents. He was doubly shocked: once to make the discovery and once again, after connecting the dots, that his asthma went away and didn't come back.[3]

Pennebaker is a key figure in all this.

He wanted to see if confronting the demon through writing worked as well as talking. When you think about it, writing comes with pretty good credentials. It's private. You don't have to show it to anyone. You don't have to *trust* anyone else with your deep dark secrets so it's a lot easier to tell the truth. Writing utilizes a different neurological pathway than speech, moving from the brain directly to the hand, which bypasses the usual inhibitions of speech with its social constraints to be polite or politically correct. And, importantly, there is something organic to writing that insists upon truth-telling. Writing doesn't work well as literature unless you feed it large doses of truth. I lead writing workshops all over the country. Occasionally we'll see a poem which starts out working really well, good music, nice metaphors. Then suddenly it hits a snag where it just falls apart: the line length goes out of control, music gets clunky, similes fall flat. If you look closely, that is precisely the point where the poet has lost courage to go into the center of a difficult truth. Ingrained into the genome of writing itself are mechanisms that will make it beautiful or interesting which are the same mechanisms that are tied directly to the truth. The writing will self-destruct if you hedge or tell it lies.

I don't know if that was the thinking process Pennebaker used to make him want to experiment with writing but somehow he thought it might do the trick. So he designed a study. He took college students and divided them in four groups. **#1** wrote about a traumatic event. **#2** wrote about an emotional reaction to a traumatic event. **#3** wrote both about the details of the trauma and the emotional reaction. **#4** served as a control, writing about something meaningless, like making a list of objects in their bedrooms. He then looked at medical dispensary records to chronicle the frequency and severity of doctor visits and discovered that three of the groups were unchanged by the intervention. But one, group **#3**, showed a precipitous 50% drop in clinic visits following just three 20-minute sessions of writing over five days. The favorable effect lasted more than six months.[4]

It wasn't writing about the traumatic event that worked, or even about the emotional response. It was making a *connection*, a linguistic linkage between the trauma and the emotional response that proffered this property of healing.

---

3 Pennebaker, *Opening Up*, 5.

4 J. W. Pennebaker and S. K. Beal, "Confronting a traumatic event: Toward an understanding on Inhibition and Disease," *Journal of Abnormal Psychology*, 95 (1986): 274-281.

Pennebaker then demonstrated that the immune responsiveness of T cells increased following this same form of deep writing in which a connection between trauma and emotional response was made.[5] Even in patients with AIDS there was a demonstrable effect.[6] Nor was the experience for the participant especially difficult. Immediately following the writing sessions there was a sense of disturbance, a slightly depressed feeling, but this discomfort rapidly dissipated and was replaced with a sense of hubris, of self-control, a greater sense of contentment which lasted for months. Later studies demonstrated a 30% improvement in lung volume for asthmatics suffering an attack.[7]

Writing of the kind that attacks difficult issues with ruthless honesty has the power to soothe psychological disturbances, to preserve or reinforce healthy states, and to reach all the way into the immune system and strengthen it. Apparently, writing can disable the destructive connection between traumatic events and the psychic and physical diseases they produce.

So isn't this what writers are doing all the time?—diving into the forbidden, looking for connections to meaning? Think of the Symbolists, Baudelaire, Rimbaud, Mallarme—their business was to take the ugly and turn it into something beautiful.

Does the attitude or the courage of the writer matter? Pennebaker analyzed the essays of subjects in his experiments and found that a reluctance to open fully to the honest inquiry impaired the ability of the exercise to provide benefit. Contrariwise, "letting-go" was associated with a measurable improvement.[8]

He then studied the words used in these exercises to see if they mattered. The more positive words, i.e., *love, hope, benefit,* that were used, the more likely there was a positive effect. The fewer negative words, like *sorrow, frustration, hatred,* etc, the better—to a point. Both high numbers of negative words and low numbers of negative words correlated with mediocre outcomes. It is necessary, therefore, to address the negative and give it voice while seeking positive connections.[9]

---

5   J. W. Pennebaker and R. Kiecolt-Glaser, "Disclosure of traumas and immune function: Health implications for psychotherapy," *Journal of Consulting and Clinical Psychology* 56 (1988): 239–245.

6   K. J., Petrie, et al., "Effects of written emotional expression on immune function in patients with human immunodeficiency virus infection. A randomized trial," *Psychosomatic Medicine* 66 (2004): 272–275.

7   J. M. Smyth, et al., "Effects of writing about stressful experiences on symptom reduction in patients with asthma or rheumatoid arthritis. A randomized trial," *JAMA*: 281 (1999): 1304–1309.

8   Pennebaker, *Opening Up,* 44.

9   J. W. Pennebaker, T. H. Mayne, and M. E. Francis, "Linguistic predictors of adaptive bereavement," *Journal of Personality and Social Psychology* 72 (1997): 863–871.

There is an interesting parallel here. A general rule of poetry is to try to include both the positive and the negative in a single line. Balance, beauty, credibility derive from that. Poetry that is either too positive or too negative dulls the interest.

More powerful in Pennebaker's essay analysis was the effect generated by the use of cognitive words such as *cause, association, realization,* etc. The presence of these words indicated a dedicated thought process surrounding the problem which had a profound effect on outcome. And finally, and most powerful of all, was the presence of a narrative thread. That is to say, those who did a little story-telling benefited most.[10]

Story-telling. We always knew it was important, didn't we. Now science is trying to catch up.

The effect Pennebaker documented is a force that might be common to all forms of expressing emotion across inhibitions. Talking, psychotherapy, confessional booths all seem to help. The doorway we know from all this—and there may be others—is that the process of deep writing, in which a linguistic connection is made between traumatic event and emotional response, produces a healing effect.

So far we've talked about writing as an exercise. What about exposure to writing? What about reading a story or hearing a poem? Might that not share some of the same qualities and potentials as the process of writing? If language is the key then perhaps both the creation of it and the hearing of it might carry its powers.

In my first collection of short stories, "Annie's Antidote" tells of a young artist patient who suffers from ulcer disease not cured by the usual interventions.[11] It becomes necessary to do an endoscopy to assist diagnosis and treatment, but she has a morbid fear of endoscopy. To her credit she shows up for the appointment but as we are about to begin she freaks out and cannot go through with it. She sits up, tachycardic and sweating.

Situations like this cannot be forced so as we are sitting around thinking what to do next, she says, "You're a poet, aren't you?"

"Yes," I say, feeling my mind suddenly morph from the rational scientific side to the creative.

"Well maybe," she says, "I could do this if you say me a poem."

The only poem I know by heart is one of mine, so with her permission I recite:

---

10   Pennebaker, "Linguistic," 863–871.

11   David Watts, *Bedside Manners: One Doctor's Reflections on the Oddly Intimate Encounters Between Patient and Healer* (New York: Harmony Books, 2005), 97.

My son brings me a stone
and asks which star it fell from.
He is serious, so I must be careful,
even though I know it will leave him someday
and he will go on gathering, for this
is one of those moments that turns suddenly
towards you, opening
as it turns, as if we paused
on the edge of a heartbeat and then
pressed forward, conscious
of the fear that runs beside us
and how lovely it is to be with each other
in the long resilient mornings.

We were both quiet for a moment in which I wasn't sure what was happening but I knew I had done everything I could do. A moment passed and she suddenly said, "I think I can do this." And then lay down on the table. Five minutes later we were done and we found the bacteria that caused her ulcer. It was a good outcome and without the poem, it wouldn't have happened.

I don't know why the poem did what it did. Was it trust? Was it knowing the doctor had another, more sensitive side? Was it the rhythms of the poem that imitated the healthy rhythms of the body? Maybe it was transformation. Beauty is transformative wherever we find it in music, nature, children ... I don't know. But, to be sure, the poem had a therapeutic effect.

So this little story creates for us an example of a poem heard having a healing effect upon someone. By that we may conclude that both the process of writing and the listening to literature have healing qualities.

Now it is very interesting to speculate where it might go from here. How, for example, does this effect work its way out from consciousness into the tissues of the body?

As it turns out our internal systems are interconnected in complicated ways which only now are being brought to light. We know where the brain is but not the mind. The mind may actually reside in many locations and may involve not just the brain but many of the organ systems. Some believe the mind resides, in part, outside the body. Some believe the gut with its complex neural networks and its ability to remember patterns of health and disease independently of the brain confer upon it qualities of a second brain. The gut is very much involved with the immune system, making a large amount of antibodies used in defense against disease.

But now we know there is a complicated connecting network that unifies these systems, a psychosomatic network as it has been called by some.[12] The brain makes peptides that enter the endocrine system and have a very strong effect upon emotions. Endorphins. Serotonin. Dopamine. Neurotransmitters. These peptides are the biochemical manifestations of emotions. Each of the peptides has the ability to evoke chemical changes and to alter behavior and change mood states. Each peptide may evoke a unique emotional tone. The entire known group of 60–70 peptides constitutes a universal biochemical language of emotions.

As it turns out, the entire intestine is lined with peptide receptors. We literally feel emotions in our "gut." Not only that, the gut makes its own peptides, as do the spleen and lymph nodes, both traditionally part of the immune system. The way we think is connected to these peptides and therefore all our perceptions and thoughts are colored by emotions and manifested in chemistry. Even white cells make these peptides. As Candice Pert, the discoverer of many of these molecules, puts it, "white cells are bits of the brain floating around in the body."[13] Do they contribute to thinking? To emotions? Most probably. Therefore, cognition is a process that spreads throughout the body, using peptides as mediators and involving both the emotions and the immune system.

Whereas we have traditionally studied the immune system, the nervous system, and the endocrine system as three separate entities, they are more likely a single, psychosomatic network connected by these peptides, under the influence of a single family of molecular messengers.

It is easy to believe that perturbations in consciousness, especially those arising from traumas unresolved over time which build up pressure against the wall of inhibition, might easily spill over by way of these peptides into our emotions and into the very way our immune system interacts with disease.

The secret combination to the lock that binds us is language. Language gets us instantly into the core of the body where these powerful and complex interconnections live. Language in the form of truthful narratives has the power of beauty to transform, can alter the flow of things, can tune the dissonance into something harmonious to strengthen our mental and physical health.

---

12   Fritjof Capra, *The Web of Life: A New Scientific Understanding of Living Systems*, (New York: Anchor Books, 1996), 282 ff.

13   Candace Pert, "Healing Ourselves and Our Society," Presentation at Elmwood Symposium. Boston, December 9, 1989.

Lalla, the 13th century Kasmirian poet, says it this way:

> I didn't trust it for a moment
> but I drank it anyway
> the wine of my own poetry.
>
> It gave me the strength to take hold
> of the darkness and tear it down
> and cut it into little pieces.[14]

It's a powerful claim for language, to "take hold of the darkness ... and cut it into little pieces."

But we have seen the evidence.

---

14   Lalla, *Naked Song*, trans., Coleman Bark, (Athens, GA: Maypop Books, 1992), 11.

Catharine Clark-Sayles

Not Enough

It is not enough: the early quiet, its coolness.
Not enough the exquisite mornings of heat
as we lay our bodies into green, splayed and open
to the juices that rise always to sun.
The taste of blueberries, the taste of a lover's tongue:
not enough. Stars sketch themselves into constellations
never known to the Greeks and it is insufficient
that we name them: waterfall, flat tire, kitchen
table like the one where we learned the mystery
of bread. Not nearly enough. So much is gone
before we know of the need to miser moments,
to hold the ringing, buoyant silences, the crispness
of air. Even death with its dissolving and erasure
is not a grand enough gesture to hold all of this.

Bibliography

Shane was her father,
her mother was Jane Eyre,
her sister Sarah Crewe.
Eight states, nine schools
and as many cousins, aunts
and uncles as three brick-and-board
shelves would hold.

Summers floating the Mississippi
with cousins Huck and Jim,
winters tramping London streets
with Uncle Sherlock
and his sister Nancy Drew.
Red Chief was a better bratty brother
because he could be put away
on the middle shelf
between Uncle Bilbo
and second cousin Podkayne.

She was not so much a lonely child
as one living in her head
absorbing possibilities:
Momma Jane taught perseverance,
Poppa Shane knew when to stand and fight
and Sarah insisted secret princesses
would never be left unloved.

Night Call

If you are in need and it is midnight,
if I leave my bed for the cold darkness,
if I stumble on the step, drive yawning to the ER,
if the light is fluorescent and numbing
and there are cries of despair from the next bed,
I will not resent more than a little
my dream forever gone, not curse you
for the warmth cooling beneath my quilt.
I will not hold you accountable
for the missing hour of sleep.
I will love the crescent moon, the sudden deer
and the hustling skunk on my street as I return.
I will love this midnight world.
I will love my skill.
I will love your need.

Julia B. Levine

Denver, 1988

I want to tell it as the story of two lovers
meeting in a park just before winter,
a light frost crusting the fields.

I want him to appear small and forsaken
beneath the immense vault of the Rockies,
his hood pulled away from his face.

A kingdom of starlings
lifts from the nearly bare branches,
one wave of disturbance becoming another,

as he watches me run, his hands in his pockets,
and I want him frozen between doubt
and a blaze of desire.

As for those birds settling back down,
I want the last few leaves they've knocked into air
to fall as apology, an error in tense.

And even if I can't decide
whether sun kindles the lawn,
or the first snow is waiting just under the hour,

every story must happen in time. In time
his gun slips from its sheath,
presses cold to my temple.

Here, he has no language for asking,
no jacket to lay between the dirt and my face.
And because the truth is a current

that both enters and carries the story,
here the story wrestles with silence,
and here it returns as a ghost

gorging on eternity
as he shoves his gun back in his pocket,
and bends to my ear, wet lips muttering,

That's all I wanted,
his boots kicking up a clatter of birdsong,
a feather sifting dark over the trail.

Shame

If I dream myself naked on a toilet
and the door won't close,
and around me there are esteemed colleagues
beside my three daughters
and the men they one day will marry;

If they look and don't turn away,
but go on talking,
passing round a bowl of freshly picked cherries
until juice bleeds down their chins;

If I will not be allowed back into that strange window
where I once unzipped my being from my body,
so that now my body refuses to pack up
its dense presence and hungers,
its ruined macula and bonespurs,

then its evidence of noise and wound and scent,
will bind me as one among many,
and I will ask for one cherry or two—
whatever my portion allows;

I will be dreaming already
into that dark globe on my tongue,
that taste of wild, sweetened rain.

Interim Report to My Late Student

in memory of Arthur Heehler

I imagine you would have liked your wake
better than I did—
the house smelling of sawdust and poverty,
all the doors open to heat
and a pit bull wandering in at dusk
from the yard where a band stumbled towards music.

One woman was skeletal.
Another looked as if she'd spent years broke and alone,
whispering to no one in particular,
Can you tell me, what really matters in the end?
Even in the simplest world
asking a question is harder than you think.

Like your best friend, Bob, one hand covering his mouth
wondering if I knew that in your last year
your bones were powder, small explosions
breaking like a meteor shower inside your body.
By then, some of the men had gathered,
holding beers and nodding.

Nights hot as this, Kevin said,
he'd bring his tripod and stay up all night
taking pictures of the tracks behind his trailer.

I gave Bob a ride home in the back seat,
his shoes held together with duct tape,
his head bowed so that no one would know it was him.
He said that you believed the dead slept
like railroad tracks, their ribs pressed up against the earth.

We were silent then, reverent almost
in the transit of bodies from one place to another.
Neither of us mentioned how we believed you
were at it again, only this time with Vicodin and Darvocet.
Or why none of us ever paid for you to see a doctor.

Forgive me. If it was a real question,
I'd have to let the answer be something
I didn't want to know.

Meg Newman

Excerpt from *Memoir*

A scrub jay darts out from underneath the maple tree and emerges onto the peak of the adjacent cherry tree. He flaps his indigo and royal blue tail feathers in unison, shakes his head north, south, west and swivels one-hundred and eighty degrees to glower with his puffed up chest toward the east. A moment later another scrub jay drives out of the maple, down to the garden, and with a zig and a zag, retreats back to the tree carrying a thin, long twig. The male, distinguished by the narrow white stripe over his eyes, surveys the land for new predators and, once satisfied, zips under the dripping mass of green leaves.

I realize I have been mesmerized and have not moved since this display began. I begin to water jog slowly, and quickly reach a consistent rhythm. The clear warm water laps around me and seeps in and out of my floatation devices as I scan the theatre, my yard, for more action to observe. This scenario would repeat many times over the next four days as the jays built their nest and I did PT in my tiny therapy pool. On good days, I notice these events as invitations to breathe deeply, marvel at the mystery and feel the beauty in my life.

Because of the nest, my partner Sherry and I decide to put off pruning the maple tree until forever, and I cease my annual rumination on how the maple's flowing leaves shade our vegetable bed. Finding the bird's nest precipitates a full cure, though not the one we have been waiting for.

On a late afternoon after I watch both the adult birds fly out, I look to see if a nest really exists. I still have delusions, but I learn that the scrub jay nest is not one of them. It is tightly woven with deep and steep walls and sits firmly between hugging branches. I wonder if the eggs are already laid and if the 16–19 day incubation period has begun. Scrub Jays are altricial: once their eggs hatch, the young birds stay in the nest for the next 18 days or so. They are born void of feathers, dependent and unable to move much. As I read this information in my dog-eared bird book, while lying flat on my bed, a sweeping shadow crosses my mind's eye. An hour later, still in the same position, I understand the shadow's message. I have something in common with these baby birds. I am void of feathers, I am unable to move much, and I am dependent, much more than I can accept at this stage of my fifty-five year old life.

Nine years ago the dominant form of art in my life was movement. Weaving on ice skates and stick handling with a puck were the brush strokes of my paintings. When I ran, making unusual strides and shifts to accommodate the terrain, I heard jazz loud and clear. My college basketball team was sometimes a well-choreographed and fast-paced ballet. Movement was how I reached calm, found balance and experienced joy. It took a single moment on an otherwise remarkably normal day to interrupt this artistry and introduce me to a new and more complicated relationship with my body, with balance, and with joy.

The house was still and cold at 5:30 AM and the wood floors creaked as I walked to the kitchen. It was the last Friday in April, 2002. I sat down to my bowl of hot oatmeal with almonds, flax and apple and readied myself for work. As a doctor at the UCSF AIDS Clinic at San Francisco General Hospital, I took care of patients with HIV/AIDS, collaborated with them on their own healing journeys, taught and mentored as much as possible and did my share of administration. I worked with uplifting and brilliant people, surrounded by exciting ideas, exchanges and compelling projects, all day and often into the night. I felt deeply content, inspired daily to be the best doctor and teacher I could be. My work offered an abundant opportunity for both service and science; I had long found my calling, my colleagues, and my professional home.

By 6:30 that evening I managed to have all patient matters tucked in and I decided to spring loose from my ever expanding pile of work. I rode my bicycle to the yoga studio and arrived in time to slip into place just before the class began. Sherry's face lit up when I arrived, and then she gave me her very seductive wink. I lit up and winked back with far less acumen but equal intention. After a few deep breaths I felt my pulse come down. I radiated heat and sweat from the bike ride; I was warm and ready to begin. A substitute emerged, saying that our beloved instructor Margaret was not well that day. The fifteen regulars exhaled a disappointed murmur.

I stretched upward with a deep breath, then my chest expanded symmetrically and my arms splayed downwards as I released the air. By the time the class was half over, I could see that the sub was visibly frustrated with my limited skill and how I modified multiple positions to avoid the torn cartilage in my left knee from locking. But I was having fun, so I moved to be out of her visual field. From the very back of the room, I enjoyed observing Sherry's graceful moves, lean spine, and her strong arms. I bent toward my toes and unexpectantly felt a flash of pressure in my spine and thick, dense heat marching down my lumbar spine and left leg. I lay down in the back of the class, my mouth and my face contorted as I silently but strenuously cried "NO!" Sherry sensed something was off and came back to check in with me—and instantly sensed something was wrong. Sherry put my bike on the rack and packed me into a flattened front seat. On the short drive home I told her that I didn't think I would ever be going to another yoga class.

Discordant notes of wrenching back and buttock pain, severe spasms, electric shocks, burning nerve pain and muscle weakness joined my somatic lexicon that very weekend. I didn't know for certain which anatomical part I had injured in my spine, but I did sense that something big had shifted and I feared nothing would ever be the same in my life.

One of my favorite teaching axioms has always been, "Denial is the most powerful physiologic mechanism." Despite the worsening pain, I decided to delude myself into believing that I would be better within a week or two, and continued conservative treatment with physical therapy. My symptoms worsened significantly; two months dragged by and we realized we needed to take a deeper look and understand more about this "injury." I then entered the spinal industrial complex, and a new patient was born.

The first four years, I remained outwardly confident and inwardly questioned whether we would be successful in restoring me to my pre-injury state, or somewhere proximal to it. Having turned to orthopedic science previously for a hand fracture, a troublesome accessory foot bone that had become injured, and the repair of two knees with torn cartilage, I had the perception that with a knowledgeable doctor, things would go well. I underestimated the treatment complexities of spinal problems even though I knew them well: A small irony was that I had been teaching the UCSF medical students and residents about the diagnosis and management of spine disease since 1996. I forgot, of course, that denial is the most powerful physiologic mechanism, especially when the medical issue is your own.

The hot sun pushed through my living room window and transported enough bright light to warm the pale yellow walls into a safe, golden yellow afternoon den. Up until then, I had only observed this serene and peaceful transition on a weekend, but here I was on a Wednesday afternoon, recovering from a discectomy, my first spinal surgery. I had finally found a position that was tolerable and I was dreamily debating with myself about whether I should get up and go to the bathroom or just stay and relish in my new found position. In that moment, I absorbed how suffering people might lie down in the snow and slowly convince themselves to stay and die happily. Everyone was at work except me and Allicat, and she, being a cat's cat, actually thought that I was home solely because she preferred it that way.

After the discectomy, I recovered quickly, and returned to work in twenty-eight days. For the next ten months I rehabbed with ferocious passion and developed an even stronger core. But, here's the thing: I still couldn't sit very long without serious pain in my spine and electric agony down my left leg. The sitting problem worsened and then another part of my spine became affected, manifested painful symptoms, and then progressed. No doubt about it—I was back in spinal hell. As before the discectomy, I sought help, I researched my options thoroughly, consulted widely, debated and questioned all treatments. This entire scenario would repeat, multiple times, over the next eight years, as my functional status declined.

It was a sunny and warm day, early in the spring, and mounds of snow were melting around the edges of a mountain meadow. Here I was; I felt wonderful. I was in my favorite black running shorts so I started running fast. I noticed that I had no pain, and I ran faster. Still no pain. I became giddy and felt so comfortable that I sprinted through the center of the meadow. Toward the end of the meadow, I lifted off the ground, flying a few inches above the meadow's fragile floor. I awoke to Allicat's inverted claw gently stroking my cheek. I was confused and then desperately sad to be back in my hurting body. I tasted the dream all day, clung to it in my less busy moments while washing my hands and stethoscope between patients.

Everything in my life felt threatened—my happy marriage, my content professional world, my sense of humor and, of course, my physicality. I vacillated between the raw anguish of the reality and my desire to place it all directly into my denial/suppression file.

Though I'd been able to return to work, I now did all my work standing, including while talking to my patients, and I regularly apologized for standing while they sat. I missed being at eye level, and they did, too. However, over time, something shifted in the exam room. Although my patients had always experienced my compassion and love for them, they now saw me as vulnerable, despite my best efforts to hide, deny, and minimize my symptoms. My patients could see my spinal disease and identified that we were both experiencing pain and illness. I had joined them in the universe of suffering, and our relationship was enhanced by it. In an unspoken way, my illness dissolved a boundary between us.

As my spinal disease progressed, I could do less and less. After eight years I wasn't able to drive, I couldn't sit more than twenty to thirty minutes a day, I couldn't stand up for longer than ten to fifteen minutes at a time, and could do so only four to five times a day. I was in a significant amount of pain, all the time. All this meant limited contact with my patients, work life, and the entire world outside my own house, which profoundly affected all my most significant relationships and especially Sherry.

Sherry and I have lived nearly half our lives together. As peers, athletes and activists we have loved, struggled, laughed, collaborated, hiked and guided each other through our late twenties into the middle of our fifties. We have built and solidified the love and experiences of decades into something tangible that we both come to for nourishment and refuge.

Despite the beautiful relationship I have with my wife and amazing family and friends, I still became physically isolated from work and all my familiar haunts and habits. I had always appreciated solitude and reveled in it. However, this was a lot of unplanned solitude with limited mobility, a package I know I didn't order. Over time, all of my important relationships have become savvier about how to love and laugh in this new conformation.

I now know I have a yet unnamed connective tissue disease that caused the breakdown of the cartilage tissue in both my knees as well as the five discs of my lumbar spine and some in my thoracic and cervical spine. Both the cartilage and the spinal discs normally have a great deal of collagen; they both function to separate and protect the bones above and below them and permit safe movement in the spine and knee. Most likely, some key protein in me is missing, a simple omission with profound consequences.

My feet used to anchor me to the Earth; I was fluid, lithe, athletic. All these years after that chilly quiet morning in April, 2002, I am wobbly, my feet hurt and I am prone to bumping into things. As a rule, nerves don't generally like being compressed for more than a few months; my L-5 nerve was compressed for over seven years, and now harbors an irreversible grudge that affects my left leg and the bottoms of both feet. All day I feel the current of three NYC subway lines trudging through my feet, intermittently dropping yellow sparks. The outside of my left leg and my thigh host a colony of one thousand sensory bees that sting, prick and burn without fatigue. After four spinal surgeries and much cobalt and chromium artificial disc hardware, my time spent upright has improved. With crutches to guide my feet and unload my spine, I can triple my upright and walking time and stabilize my gait. Balance is more syncopated for me now, and my movements have taken on a profoundly changed artfulness.

The inbound and outbound flight patterns around the scrub jay nest remain busy while I watch from my outdoor theatre—my therapy pool. The scrub jays have been collecting and saving food, and within the next two weeks, baby scrub jays will arrive. In the pool with my floatation devices I am freed from gravity, truly weightless and my spine is unloaded; I am thriving. I keep hoping to find more ways to suffer less. Hope is a multi-edged sword and I have been a hope-a-holic my whole life. I know the seductive benefits of hope but I knew little about hope's darker, seedier side.

During these long years, I've found that if I was just hoping and organizing to the nth degree how I would become all better, I wasn't living with reality. Living in the future, I was missing some of the more difficult moments, but I was also missing some of the joyful ones. I still do everything I can to improve my condition, but when I arrive at now, surrounded by things exactly as they are, I become most alive. The present moment is so different from what it used to be but, still, I can feel its richness; it is a nonlinear, tenuous and fluid peace that I keep renegotiating.

Larry Ruth

Friday Afternoon and Other Adventures

After the cappuccino, reading
the news, leisure, no distractions,
I've been a long time sitting, neatly
folded section of Friday afternoon,
now to walk away from *Weekend Arts*
away from the table, south, down
College Avenue, summer day, dream
to Milestone Basin, Sequoia and hike
two blocks to the car, more, going
to the fire road in the hills, muse
about that conversation at the next
table and at the corner, wait
for the signal, think about music
tonight, Coleman Barks reading
Rumi, tablas, flutes, bliss
and blues, Sufis, summer is here,
love, live a little, revival,
green light, go east, step up
step off the curb, speeds by

that first car, driver cuts the corner
too close, step back, nick of time,
but not far enough, there're two cars,
the second, burnt orange box Honda,
driver not looking at us, looking south,
the opposite direction, front of the car
right here, engine revs, soft tire treads
on my toes, wheels roll and backward
I go, somersaulting over and away,

end on the asphalt, sitting on my butt,
dazed, my foot tingling, numbs out just
before five, quitting time, next to me a man
looks down; it's Sammy, he says, "Are you …"
I don't answer, so he tries a different tack:
"Do you want me to call …" I tell him no,
I just need to get my bearings, follow
Annelise and her friend back to Strada

No second cappuccino, sit for a bit, but they
want 911, no pressure, we talk, I call my doctor,
the office is closed, "in the event of a medical emergency,
please dial 9-1-1" I don't but don't move either, until
the world slows down. Thigh throbs, walk to the car (an enemy …
I wonder), get in, drive home, and *pressure* realize my head
hurts, end up at Alta Bates Hospital, place where I was born.
Funny, though, the toe seems pretty much unaffected.
CT scan shows head, no fractures. Bob says "Get out of here."
Jessie reminds me not to *ignore the bruises. Ice and rest,
more ice and you are definitely going to be sore. And stiff.*

Next morning, still in my bathrobe, figuring out what
works and trying to get started, a police officer comes by,
someone I know, Lyle Ledward, star of the Seventh Grade class,
fastest runner, six hundred yard dash, big smile, he wants to talk.
After he gathers "just the facts," he reaches out, takes my hand
and shakes it. Via email, my friend Arpita recommends Rescue
Remedy—"helps after shocky-scary things." At Whole Foods
or Berkeley Bowl. And Arnica pills, she writes, "for the stiffness."
All this—no music   no walk in the hills   no revel—all happens.

Friday, Saturday, Sunday, not bliss, but not bad either
Sunday night at my desk, healing as writing, blessed
are the words before they are written
Monday morning
flies past.

Occupational Therapy

Months after the accident, I choose romance—
wheelbarrow, quelque *painteurs*, Provence, red
poppy, iridescence, *Coquelicot*, nineteen seventy-two,
Aix, the white-bearded guy passing for Paul Cezanne,
scrounging dans le Cours Mirabeau, geography
of the moment, places I hadn't thought of in years
instead of answering her question—
                    "What do you want?"

Tired of good wishes, self-congratulations
for having survived, stumbling
over some revelation I couldn't grasp, think
elsewhere, flood tides, turquoise
spiral of wave and kelp blossom, songs of the real
instead of impressions of what I'd wanted.
Replace *lost* with *found*.

Maybe she was right. After all *time present and time past*,
I'd already lost the present at least once. First time.
For fifteen minutes, I try to answer her questions
& remember that moving pencil across paper
is a big part of it, then stop, exhausted,
but like it, want to write again.

Second go. Since   *what's present now will later be past*
for a trial period, I try to write the future. Look at printed words
for ideas, trace one, *apprehension*, think but can't make out
what it means, can't recognize any real difference between
apprehension and *asparagus*

Picked up the notebook later, looked,
found nothing, no future, my time
apparently spent writing in the sand
and proofreading blank pages on the way
to Mont Saint Victoire, Sisteron, and Gap.

Casting a Spell: *Summer*

Change something, exactly what doesn't matter,
new or old, who or what doesn't matter, conjure now,
make vivid, believe it alive
                    as one body enfolds
another, awaken to an alarm clock shift of her body,
one whom you love, had forgotten you loved,
met again on a summer's day, Sierra
granite and glaciers, measuring time
in the careless crush of her arms.

Each day, cross the river, twenty-minutes more
or less, swim, whisk yourselves dry, reverie
and rhyolite giving off warmth, hike to happiness,
long days cool into evening, weaving sunset
and sleep, dreaming of
                    talus, slopes and scree
to Old Army Pass, big rock, the back country,
bighorn sheep, ewes and calves at Soldier Lake,
corn lilies and columbine in bloom, purple
onions below at Rock Creek,
                    old avalanches
mark the trail to foxtail pines, to the saddle
at Guyot, then down, a long, sandy traverse
to Crabtree Meadows
                    ford the creek, veer east,
take the fisherman's trail, uphill to the meadows
and lakes, boulders bright with snow, sliding
toward solid ground, to the water beneath the cliff.
Walk on, to the shore of a lake
                    high, blue and deep,

remember that day of fishing and laughter,
the creek's outlet silver, golden, going scarlet
with a thousand spawning trout.

Next morning, follow the shore of Guitar Lake,
climb seventy-odd switchbacks to the crest,
cross over, off trail long way round,
scramble through Whitney Pass and down
or linger at the top before leaving, bend
                    day and night

and day, flow, river carving curves in the rock,
decades unchanging even as it changes,
never the same water, not the same
time.
      Find your pack. Call her, say, "*Let's go, leave
for Lone Pine, hike from Horse Corral, Cottonwood,
any trail, just two of us …*
                    Afternoons and asters,
snowmelt trickling down the rock.

Veneta Masson

Silence and Other Lessons from the Language of Music

Why did I say yes? I'd just heard myself accept David Watts's invitation to join the poetry faculty of The Healing Art of Writing—2010. "We expect the faculty to be writing, too," he added, "right along with the participants."

"Ah!" I may have said by way of acknowledgment, but I was doubtful. The plain truth was that I wasn't writing. I was in a silent season—a long silent season!

But wait a minute, I thought after hanging up the phone. I haven't been completely silent. For the past eleven years, I've been studying jazz piano and making music. When I began, Ron Elliston, my teacher, told me straight out that he couldn't teach me to play by ear, improvise or master jazz. What he could do is teach me the language of music and help me to make it my own. Good enough, I decided. I'm in.

At my piano lesson a few days before David's call, I played a tune I'd been working on. Ron's critique surprised me. "I don't hear the silence," he said. "Silence is as much a part of music as sound. It's what gives sound its meaning. And remember, just as the vocalist and horn player have to breathe, so do you, so does the listener."

I asked myself how that take-home message might apply to writing as well. My imagination began to play with the theme of creative silence and, soon enough, other memories about how my explorations in music have informed my poetry began to surface. I knew very quickly that these lessons were what I wanted to share with you in my talk about craft. Here they are, translated into what I hope is practical advice for writers.

1.   Silence gives meaning to sound.

I was fortunate in my beginnings as a poet—somewhat late, in my thirties. I'd joined a church whose structures included a daily hour of quiet meditation, weekly spiritual reports, and annual silent retreats, all this at a time in my life when I was immersed in my 24-7 responsibility for the care of patients and staff (I was nurse practitioner and director) in a busy inner-city clinic where crises seemed to occur daily. I found myself spilling the remains of those chaotic days into a journal during my evening quiet hour.

Over time, some of the people and events I had written about began to turn into poems, often untraceable to whatever jotting inspired them. We began to include some of these in our clinic's annual reports along with photos, drawings and writings from my workmates. As the financial and statistical data our non-profit corporation was required to publish each year got squeezed into a couple of pages at the end, we realized that what we were producing looked more like a corporate journal.

Because these offerings had been well received by our friends and contributors, I decided to mark Community Medical Care's fifteenth anniversary (and raise some funds) by publishing a chapbook of my poems accompanied by evocative portraits of several of our patients taken by Jim Hall, our founder and physician. Marc Pekala, a graphic design student at American University, designed it as his senior project. With financial backing from a few sponsors, we mustered the courage to print a thousand copies which we sent to our supporters, gave as gifts, or sold.

I'm convinced that none of this would have happened without my commitment to daily quiet time. As the poet David Whyte wrote in his book *Crossing the Unknown Sea*, "Without silence, work is not music, but a mechanical hum, like an old refrigerator...only noticed ...when it finally brings itself to a stop."

I became serious about my vocation and wanted to master the poet's craft. So I attended a series of poetry workshops at our local writer's center. These taught me a great deal about how poems are made and perfected, but it was my spiritual practice of silence that allowed me the space and time to continue to dredge up poems from the mulch heap of my imagination and life experience. Regular silent retreats, in which participants are instructed not to work or specifically direct their energies, have helped me to welcome rather than dread the seasons in which my poetic voice is silent. It's all part of the cycle of renewal.

I've learned that poems, like people, don't mature overnight. The journey from journal or scrap paper to finished poem can take years—and for some that journey will never be completed. I've also come to value the way a poem breathes with help from phrasing, punctuation, line breaks, and white space on the page. When spoken aloud, I believe that a poem deserves to be framed in silence so that poet and listener can focus before and reflect after the reading. These seconds of silence can set the tone and may convey as much meaning as the words themselves.

2. To become a good player, you have to be an educated listener.

I notice that there are always musicians in the audience when I go out to listen to jazz. I'm not talking only about amateurs. I'm talking about the pros. Sure, there is an element of rivalry in their attentiveness, but I've learned that they're also thinking about which tunes are being played, which musicians they'd like a chance to perform with or cop a lesson from, and what new riffs or chord changes they can "steal" for themselves.

Jazz musicians know that you can't play improvised music if you don't have hundreds of the tunes called standards locked into memory, ready to be called up at a moment's notice. They also have to be able to hear not only what they are playing but what others in the combo are playing in the same moment. It's this sense of tradition and community that creates the synergy needed to keep the music alive and thriving.

Reading and listening to poetry are also fundamental to the poet's art. Think of the bearers of oral tradition through the centuries—the West African griot, the British and Celtic bards, the itinerant poets of today who draw crowds in schools, libraries and auditoriums, even stadiums. This contemporary lot includes artists as diverse as rapper Snoop Dogg, British poet and performer David Whyte, and the poet in residence at a local school or hospital.

I didn't have any consistent guidance in my own literary education. From my English and lit classics classes in high school, I went straight into the technical nursing program at a community college. When I had a chance to pick up some arts and humanities courses later on, I chose French and German literature, out of curiosity. My knowledge of English and American literature is still patchy, but it makes the journey of discovery all the more fascinating.

That said, I'm pleased to report that I have in my possession a few books of poetry over fifty years old, books that I've read and packed, stored and unpacked numerous times. Except for *Sound and Sense*, a high school anthology I've held onto ever since, I'm not sure how or why I acquired them—but they convince me that I was drawn to poetry at least by age sixteen.

I remember clearly that, at twenty-two, I first read "Strokes" by William Stafford on my commute across the Bay Bridge from Berkeley to San Francisco while working on my bachelor's degree in nursing. I still remember being struck by the opening line, "The left side of her world is gone…" I was already a registered nurse and thought that the care of stroke patients held no mystery for me. But that poem opened a door to understanding that I hadn't even realized was there.

A few years later, I was a visiting nurse driving long distances between patients' homes without so much as a radio or tape player in the car. To keep myself occupied, I began memorizing poems that I taped up on the dashboard. I'd heard a story about a political prisoner in solitary confinement for years who was forbidden even books and relied on memorized poems and passages of scripture to endure the isolation. If that ever happened to me, thought, I want to be prepared! Where did those dashboard poems come from? Looking back through my old high school anthology in preparation for this talk, I discovered many of them.

With Ron's prodding, I work as hard as I can to memorize the music I want to play because, as he says, you can't be stuck on the page and still bring a tune to life or open to the flow of inspiration you need to improvise. I want to do the same with the poems that are important to me—give them a permanent place in my mind and heart where they can inspire, inform and nurture.

3.   Trapped in thought, you cannot groove.

That's how jazz pianist and educator Kenny Werner says it in *Effortless Mastery*, a book I keep going back to for its practical wisdom. My teacher Ron puts it another way. When I ask him how he's able to play long melodic lines that can go on for minutes—and still hold listeners' attention—he says simply, "Don't think." To be sure, while not thinking he is drawing on a lifetime of experience as a musician as well as mastery of technique and theory. But great artists of all kinds rely on their ability to tap into what jazz icon Bill Evans called the universal mind, the unfettered flow of creativity. I've heard it called being in "the space." While some have used drugs to try to achieve release into that space, it's a dangerous and unreliable path that may lead nowhere.

To free my own imagination, I often draw on my experiences of guided imagery. After my younger sister died, I remember trying to come to terms with her death. Certainly I was comfortable in my professional role as nurse and had shepherded many patients and families through the passage from life to death, but it had never come so close or seemed so monumental as when Rebecca died.

During this time, a friend loaned me her copy of an audiotape by Clarissa Pinkola Estes called "The Creative Fire." In it, the author and folklorist quotes an old proverb: "If *Muerte* [death] comes and sits down beside you, you are lucky, because Death has chosen to teach you something." All right, I thought. I've been lucky. What *does Muerte* have to teach me? I sat in a quiet place, closed my eyes, and waited for the empty "screen" inside my mind to fill with whatever image would present itself. That encounter was what gave rise to my poem "*La Muerte.*" In the original first line, lopped off early on, I am surprised to discover that Death is not the "dark, rapacious male" I had expected to meet. Quite the opposite. Here are the first lines from that poem, which taught me so much:

> Old Mother Death sits
> down beside me.
> Neither cruel nor kind
> she does not take, she receives.
> We are, all of us, her wards...

4.   Structure ignites spontaneity. Limits yield intensity.

Credit for these words goes to Stephen Nachmanovitch in his book *Free Play— Improvisation in Life and Art*. Even jazz improvisation isn't just free play. It has a structure. When you improvise, you work within the framework of the tune you are "playing on." The style (bebop, ballad or bossa nova, for example), tempo, number of bars, key signature, and chord progressions are givens. The fun begins when you deconstruct the melody, rhythm, and chords and "play off" them or substitute your own.

Poets today generally don't write in traditional forms such as the sonnet, sestina, or triolet. But when I have experimented with them, I've been gratified to discover that the "rules" take me to places I might not have gone otherwise. Because I need a rhyming word, a particular rhythm, or a specific number of lines, I may write a different poem than I anticipated. Occasionally it makes for a thrilling ride.

Even without a fixed form, an ad hoc structure seems to emerge from the sounds or content I'm working with. I worked hard but enjoyed making what I think of as a three-in-one poem, "Fortune." The idea is that you can read the two columns either down or across, rather like a crossword puzzle. When I started, I knew only that I wanted to write about my devotion to fortune cookies and see what kind of poem might emerge by combining a few of the fortunes that have come my way in Chinese restaurants.

Fortune

1.	A journey must begin	Yes, let it begin
	with a single step	the sacramental breaking of cookie
2.	Don't be afraid to	trust the tiny article of faith inside
	take that big step	find riches, fame, romance
3.	If you can't decide	let fortune guide you
	up or down	to the edge of reason
	try moving across	that beguiling divide
4.	Many a false step	full of portent
	is made by standing still	jump

5. Music has its origin in natural sound; poetry has its origin in music.
Kenny Werner writes that "language is the retention of rhythm without pitch—in this way, poetry was born of music. Distilling poetry of its rhythm, we have prose." And think about this: the word music derives from muse—the Greek name given to those mythical sisters who inspire the creation of literature and the arts. So look for music in the poems you write.

There's something deep inside each of us that resonates with strong rhythms—probably because they echo the heartbeat. Rhyme and other forms of consonance and repetition also get our attention. There's simple chant, usually one short phrase that you repeat over and over. The standard American song has its share of repetition, too. It's an A-A-B-A form, which means that the first melody repeats twice, is interrupted by a second melody (the "bridge"), then repeats a third time. Lyrics that may not be eloquent are memorable because of their rhythm, rhyme, and fusion with the melody or rhythm. I suspect that's why it's a snatch of music rather than poetry or prose that gets stuck in our head and repeats endlessly, sometimes for days.

Think about rap—rhymed lyrics performed in time to a beat. Without the instrumental or synthesized beat, you have spoken word poetry. You may not find it in literary magazines or anthologies, but it has a long tradition and undeniable appeal to a broad swath of the population. The level of creativity and craftsmanship are often high.

I only attempted something like rap once—a poem called "Cheers for Bobby" inspired by the rhyming "cheers" chanted by the girls jumping rope on the sidewalks of the clinic neighborhood to set and keep their rhythm. Mine started out like this:

> One infection
> Two infections
> Three infections
> Four
> Floxin
> Doxy
> Penicillin
> More...

Okay, this excerpt doesn't fare well on the page, so get yourself a jump rope and try chanting it. The sound of my poetry has to satisfy my listening ear when I speak it aloud. I may not use end rhyme or a fixed rhythm but I want to hear music in the condensed, high voltage language of a poem.

6. My music and yours may differ—there's a whole world of music out there.

Kids for sure and most adults have a fierce loyalty to what they call "my music." They can hum the tune, beat out the rhythm and, if there are words, they know them by heart. This music cements friendships, energizes the weary, helps to mend broken hearts, offers solace to the beaten down, companionship to the lonely, and sheer gratification to the music lover. Whether it's country, folk, blues, gospel, pop or opera, it's powerful stuff.

And poetry? Do we allow ourselves to name and claim our favorite kind of poetry, our favorite poets? I've heard it said that poetry is beyond category and should only be judged good or bad. I disagree. For myself, I like what I think of as working poems. They are accessible but rich in metaphor and sound. They enlighten, teach, heal, challenge, amuse, or offer me a new perspective on something I'd already formed an opinion about. They stay with me and don't get old. Other people like poetry that uses language in unusual ways, or follows a stream of consciousness wherever it might lead. I have friends who like the classics—formal poems that have stood the test of time. Others gravitate to poems that tell a story.

I don't take offense when someone says, "I don't like poetry" or "I have no use for it." But I wonder if it's a question of limited exposure. If you don't find anything you like in *Poetry* or *The New Yorker,* I want to say, what about Garrison Keillor's anthology *Good Poems* or the weekly poem Ted Kooser presents in his online column *American Life in Poetry*?

Not long ago, an acquaintance with whom I was chatting about some of the poets whose work is important to me, leaned forward and exclaimed, "Doctors write poetry? Nurses? I can't imagine it!" Yes, clinicians write. Patients write. Family members write. A great many everyday people write. Who hasn't, in a moment of crisis or infatuation or despair, scribbled a line or two of poetry? More of us than have written a song, I would guess.

7. Having your own label is a good thing.

In the music world, having your own label is something to be celebrated, not questioned as it still is in some literary circles. Everyone from pop stars to the local jazz artists I go to hear seems to have their own label. I have my own imprint, too: Sage Femme Press. Technology makes it feasible and increasingly affordable. I'm no salesman—I haven't the temperament for it—but I do know this: whether it's a book, a single poem published on a postcard, or a website, I want to present my work in a personal way. And I want more than my words to speak for me. I am grateful for every opportunity I've had to collaborate with artists, photographers, and graphic designers and to put our collaborative work directly into the hands of those for whom it was intended. Even if the "those" come down to just one person! It's not sales volume that counts. As Wikipedia (our collaborative online encyclopedia) tells us, "communication is a process whereby information is enclosed in a package and is channeled and imparted by a sender to a receiver via some medium…All forms of communication require a sender, a message, and an intended recipient…" In other words, my vocation or call as poet is only fulfilled if my poems (the little packets of meaning I have lovingly and laboriously created) are received.

In closing, I want to leave you with some food for thought from Kenny Werner: "Once I was asked, 'What is the next stage of evolution in music for the next century?'

My answer was that the evolution of music is not the issue. It is the evolution of the musician that's most important. The artist must take his rightful place in society as a teacher, metaphysician, and visionary." Does that apply to those of us who practice the healing art of writing? I say yes.

Mary Stone

Dystonia

We try to read the opaque slant of afternoon light
I'll make the first guess: seeds?
You make the second guess: smoke?
Reds shift to yellows, the whole spectrum
turns on its side

> *to the left, to the left*

Straighten up, please

> \\\

Let it go, please

> *to the left, to the left*

The neurologist laughs
singing his daughter's favorite song

> *to the left, to the left*

He wears Italian loafers, starched shirt, tie

Left Sternocleidomastoid
  Left Splenius capitus
    Left Scalene
      Left Levator scapulae

He injects toxin only on Tuesdays

                    \\\

Screw the head
Unscrew the head
Straighten up, please

                    \\\

Wheels crunch on gravel
hot stars shoot
blues shift to violets, the whole spectrum
turns on its side.

Wildfires Are Following Me Around

Four wildfires in three weeks:
this is no confession, but
my aura is extremely red,
even the landscape suffers.

I'm warning you
to douse yourself
or better yet, stay away.

The clairvoyant says
to think blue thoughts,
apply color wheel theory,

avoid cigarettes,
airplanes, lovers,
children, mirrors

everything inflammable.

How Do Old Women Pray?

My children are fed, thank you.

God, your silence troubles me.

~~~~~~

I am no athlete
anymore,
no yogini
with supple spine
and bendy hips –
send me
a noisy psalm
clattering in the trees.

~~~~~~

Moss-softened oak branches
pray dappled old women:
Soft as moss, branched as oak, dappled as prayer.

Dapple me,
woman prays,
dapple me soft,
dapple me old,
dapple me oaken.

A woman's prayer:
for a moss-softened dappled oaken branching,
for a prayerful oldening.

Ruth Saxey-Reese

What this field cannot hold

Fog descending like wool
obscures all but the closest details:
the antlers looking away,
the firs pointing fingers.

Your breath still caught in frozen bubbles,
I hinge them on the fence for bait
clack-clacking together.

For three days, I float as if dead.
My eyes open, my shirt hangs dry,
my shirt opens, my eyes hang dry.

In the night, the old horse went down,
no one saw. In the morning
only her eyes move.
Beloved, who can bear this body.

And this is how I slow myself until you return:
each breath shallower, shallower.
If visitors come, I pretend sleep.

And when I dream your return,
you wear new skin,
peeled and luminous.
A swan is slung across your back,
its neck trailing your spine.

You lay down the blood trail
and I will meet you in the east field,
seep within each seed,
burst each dormant blade of grass.

Ask Away

First take care of bodies,
come conscious,
anxious islands each.

So the mapping, the lines
crossing and recrossing
latitudes. And what if
coordinates collide like
Pacific wrecks?

What then—chart away—
when it refuses to startle
us anymore, let's shut up finally
and ask the price of sky.
The heaviest sky,

becalmed.

This ferry of days
seeking mooring,
a lucent beaching, no doubt.

Zoomorphic

We live as a pack,
roam together
from room to room,
watch each
eye flick,
hair raise,
nail click.

Closing doors
not allowed.
Nosing is,
and growling at treats taken.

Night is synched breath,
curved spines,
twitching muscles in the chase.

The shared heat of survival.

Wendy Patrice Williams

The Autobiography Of a Sea Creature

Coming Home To My Body

Prologue

Giraffes surrounded me on the wall, those long necks. Covered by plastic, they were cold when I touched them. The smell of alcohol reminded me of the nurse who would dab my arm with a wet cotton ball and prick me with a needle. Dr. Constad's voice was warm gravel. "Look at you," he said, squatting so his eyes were at equal height with mine. "You are a miracle." Happiness filled up my little body, like air rushing into a green balloon. "Unbelievable," he continued. "I wouldn't have bet a plug nickel on you when you were a baby." The balloon burst. I was so ashamed I could hardly hear him continue. "But look at you now."

As soon as I was naked on the examining table, his hands kneaded my stomach. He dug deep, asking questions with his fingertips and palms. I stared at the ceiling, afraid. What was he looking for? He searched quickly, furiously, but methodically, bent on discovering something hard, that olive of stone, seed of death. His hands seemed determined to find any possible intruder.

"I don't feel anything hard," Dr. Constad pronounced. "Nice and soft."

"Will she have trouble with her stomach later, say when she's fifty?" my mother once asked Dr. Constad after the examination.

"She shouldn't," he answered. "We'll keep checking, of course."

I had no idea what fifty meant. I was not yet two when I started to worry.

Horseshoe Crabs

In records from my hospitalization after my suicide attempt at age twenty-two, I found the familiar phrase twenty-six days old. My mother had told the social worker about the operation that I had undergone as an infant. He wrote no special note to follow up on this information. The rest of the report focused on my thyroid gland and the irregularity of my periods. Blood had been drawn, a gynecology exam administered. Hormones, or female problems, had contributed to my admittance to the hospital, the notes conclude. My cold turkey withdrawal from Valium prescribed for a TMJ (tempero-mandibular joint) problem—the actual precipitating factor of my breakdown—was not something that I would have mentioned at the time. After all, according to the dentist, Valium was just like aspirin.

The notes refer to my one brief meeting with the psychiatrist and his prescription for anti-depressants and to a consultation with a social worker three weeks after my admission, who wrote: *Patient advised to seek employment (want ads supplied). Patient should pursue stable family life (stipend allotted for purchase of feminine hygiene products and new clothes).*

Years later, I understood the origins of my instability. At the encouragement of my therapist, I drew the image I had of myself as a baby—a floating monster, wound round with strands of red spaghetti. A fetal body with a blue belly and blue rubbery legs, small feet webbed like a duck's. Bald, blue head and red face. Giant amber insect eyes as if on fire, the eyes windows to my insides. A gash on my belly, red and purple angry strokes. In the picture, huge hands held up as if screaming *STOP!* yet the fingers were limp, wavy as if boneless. In fact my whole body was floppy, cast adrift, given up as if flowing with a current.

This was the image of my beginnings that I carried with me—a larval creature floating in outer space. A baby who, in all likelihood, had not received anesthesia for stomach surgery at three-weeks-old. A baby who was given a muscle paralyzer. At the time, it was believed that anesthetic drugs were too dangerous for infants. Besides, they rationalized, babies did not feel pain. And if they did, they would not remember.

As a baby, I had a condition called pyloric stenosis. The muscle around the pyloric valve between the stomach and small intestine swelled and food could not pass through. This problem is more easily diagnosed nowadays and the remedy less severe, but in 1952, the obstetrician diagnosed my symptoms incorrectly and by the time I had surgery to open the passageway at twenty-six days old, I weighed only four pounds, down from six pounds, seven ounces.

I used to believe that my mother saved my life single-handedly. Her stories said as much. I pictured her as twice her size, bent over a huge medical book propped up on a lectern at the public library as she searched day after day for the cause of my illness, flipping page after page. Suddenly, she pointed to the obscure paragraph describing my symptoms: *projectile vomiting, weight loss.* "Pyloric stenosis!" she cried. She called Dr. Constad, who corroborated her diagnosis on the phone, and whisked me off to the hospital. To me, she was Supermom. A God, only more so: she gave me life twice.

Later I learned the actual story. The obstetrician caring for me, Dr. Karr, blamed my mother for my problem digesting food, saying that she was nursing me incorrectly. My mother doubted this from the beginning since she had nursed Mike, my brother, successfully. Reading a paperback written by Dr. Spock while sitting at our kitchen table, my mother noticed a paragraph describing my symptoms perfectly. Was *pyloric stenosis* the answer to the question that burned inside her? Soon after, Dr. Constad, my brother's pediatrician, actually saved my life by looking in on me during a house visit for Mike. I was twenty-six days old and weighed only four pounds. The light drained from his face, my mother told me, when he saw me in my crib. "Take her to the hospital immediately," he said.

Dead babies haunted our family. Lawrence, my mother's brother, died of a high fever at three years old. Her cousins, four infant boys, died of what was then called "summer's complaint" and later understood to be lactose intolerance. The row of small white gravestones are smooth now, the words long rubbed away. Mike was very sick as a baby. Somehow, as my mother tells the story, he was exposed to radiator fluid after she gave birth to him in the back seat of their car where my father had piled old rusty radiators. Mike recovered in an incubator. A few years later, doctors thought he had leukemia and hospitalized him. Tests revealed that he was allergic to cow's milk. Two premature babies of my mother's died ten years before Mike was born, one came during a hurricane and the other as the result of a car accident. Dead babies. Dead babies everywhere.

My mother used to tell me that back in the old days, dead babies were not buried in their own plots but placed in caskets with anonymous adults. I imagined a dead baby lying on the chest of a corpse and oddly sensed the weight of this baby on my chest each night before bed, my breath shallow. I had come to think of it as a giant moth wrapped up, like a mummy, as though a spider had seized her—a dead baby wound round in bandages, bound by tubes like spaghetti red with tomato sauce, roping in and out of every opening like worms. *You looked like an alien being, a creature from outer space*—my mother's words, the way she described me hundreds of times during my life. Not even a baby, dead or alive.

Once I dreamed that my mother and I stared into a toilet at what looked like a slab of meat in the bowl. What to do with it, we wondered.

"Stuff it down," my mother said, "it'll go."

"It'll clog the pipes," I said. "It won't fit."

My mother flushed anyway. The bowl filled with churning water and overflowed. It wouldn't go down, but she kept trying.

The day after I was admitted to the hospital, my mother waited near a single sterile room where the nurses would bring me after surgery. She had arrived early to the ward, after sending dad to work and Mike to Aunt Terry's, only to find that I had been whisked away to surgery hours earlier. I was failing, the staff told her—no time for signing consents.

"That was the darkest hour of my life," my mother said. "I paced the hallway, stood at the window and watched people below, rushing by on Chancellor Avenue. I wanted to be one of them with regular cares. I remember every thought as if my mind were a movie camera."

After the operation, the nurses wheeled me into my hospital room. My mother said they did not speak to her as she stood in the hallway and waited while they settled me. No one ever came back out to offer a word of support or explain how the operation went. "A tiny lump wrapped in black hoses, the diameter of a quarter," went my mother's incantation. "You looked like an alien. Even so, I wished I could pick you up and hold you, but I wasn't allowed in. Besides, you were too fragile, the tubes too big."

I was laid into a crib enclosed by an oxygen tent and pushed near the observation window so that my mother could see me from the hallway. She told me later how the nurses fed me with something that looked like a large syringe. I always imagined it to be like a turkey baster. She thought they were injecting the food into my spine, which horrified her. Later I learned that the nurses likely pushed the food into my stomach via a feeding tube. Day and night, the nurses observed me through a large window in the wall opposite. "It seemed like a room made of glass," as my mother described it.

My mother made sure she was beside me at the window every morning at 6:00 AM, "I'd wake up and look at that empty crib beside me," she said. "It motivated me. Be assured, when there's a crib at home without a baby in it, that baby is at death's door."

I began to gain weight. The surgeon met with my mother when I was ready to go home from the hospital. I was just under two months old. He told her in what my mother called "thick German," that my survival hinged on her ability to keep me from crying. "Mrs. Villiams," he said, "vee vill not be doing surgery again." There were two sets of stitches, she understood, one around the pylorus valve, between the stomach and small intestine, and a second set closing my abdomen. If I cried, he explained, the stitches would likely burst and I would die.

My mother was grim. That night she huddled with my father, and they drew up a battle plan. During the day while he was at work, she would stand watch, picking me up the second I started crying. In the evening, my father would stand guard while she cooked and cleaned up. They would arrange for my brother to spend the next month at my aunt and uncle's, so they could focus undistracted. The war was on.

"Your dad and I worked as a team," my mother told me—one of the few positive comments she'd ever made about this difficult time. On weekends, they put me out in a bassinet in front of the fireplace for visitors to see. "We were very proud of you, you know."

She went on to remark about my brother's response to the attention I got. "You had a distinctive way of crying, a kind of subdued whimper," she went on, and Mike learned it. When company sat around the living room, oohing and ahhing over you in the bassinet, Mike stood in the middle of the room, imitating your cries—'hew, hew'—his face screwed up with fake tears. It was the oddest thing." Looking back, what seems odd is the fact that my mother didn't have a clue as to why her son was behaving that way.

I healed very quickly from the operation. Each night, my mother tucked me into a bassinet beside her bed, calling me her little sea turtle and sometimes, her little dove. She said that she would wake up, and I'd be just lying there happily cooing. After those first few months home from the hospital, I was "no trouble," a delight—a good, quiet baby who could play for hours alone in my crib, pretending to read the books that she had given me. Mike was a "handful." He was allergic to milk, as yet undiagnosed. "Of course, Mike's stomach must have been bothering him terribly," she added guiltily.

And yes, I was very, very good. There was a bad baby inside me though—the burden baby who was still broken. Later, a recurring childhood nightmare would haunt me of a brick dislodging from the edge of a hole in the foundation of a building, scattering thick dust that lingered ominously in the air. I'd wake up sweating, my heart racing, fearing that at any moment, the house would collapse.

By surviving the operation, I grew up believing that I had cheated death. By living, I was thumbing my nose at the Creator. God had wanted me to die, and I had disobeyed.

"*You* birthed me," I remember blaming my mother when I was a teenager after she had criticized my dirty room.

"Yes, I did, didn't I?" she reflected, pausing in her vacuuming, holding the attachment perfectly still in the air between us, and tilting her head inquiringly as she contemplated this fact. She smiled mischievously, delighted with her discovery. "It certainly is my fault, yes. I can't deny it—I birthed you." We both laughed, but underneath my accusation, I was searching for the answer to an unasked question. I remember her once saying, "Even though you had a stomach problem, I felt lucky to have a girl." *Even though.*

Those early days after I arrived home from the hospital were hard on my three-year-old brother. Each morning, he headed for the street corner and kicked the curb near the sewer. Just kicked and kicked. When Dr. Constad arrived for a home visit to check me, he asked my mother why Mike was sitting alone on the curb down the street. She told him that she was so busy caring for me, she had no time for him. "If you don't pay that poor kid some attention, he's going to grow up with a huge hatred." The doctor's observation confirmed my parents' decision to ship him off to Uncle Harold and Aunt Helen's for several weeks. There is a photo of my brother and me posed in front of the Christmas tree years later. He is behind me, hoisting a toy rifle, a look of anger darkening his face. I look distracted as I push a baby doll stroller with large black-gloved hands, my eyes cast to the side, my face solemn. His rage and my guilt, a division driven between us by circumstances over which we had no control. A division continuing into adulthood.

A milestone photo was taken of Dad and me when I made it to one year old—a close-up photo of our faces, his close to mine. He is a beaming full moon. Scrubbed and clean, he glows happily, his eyes smiling. I am happy, too, smiling what my mother calls a classic "buttermilk smile," no teeth but lips upturned. In front of us is a huge sheet cake and a mushroom candle at the center with a white shaft and a red cap with white polka dots. We celebrated. I had made it out of the danger zone.

In kindergarten, I sat by myself at snack time, just my milk and me. I focused on the red and white carton. The waxiness of its surface. How it was shaped like a little house. The pile of bubbles floating on the milk's surface. I was intent on sucking up the rich white liquid through a straw and making sure I did not make a slurping noise when I got to the bottom. Every snack time was the same—the red carton and me.

Miss Anderson invited my mother in to speak with her. Why was I so shy, she wanted to know. After my mother told her about my operation, she made me sit with the same group of three children during snack and lunchtime. Slowly, I began to play with others in the playhouse and in the sandbox. I wouldn't push my toy truck in the circle with the other children while the sounds of honking horns played on the phonograph, but I did begin to assert myself. When Miss Anderson asked who wanted to play the sandpaper blocks with the "orchestra" during music time, I raised my hand.

Suzanne Tay-Kelley

Gangsta Holiday

Braddah's so chillin', he's in his element
    grim cover's busted, bares mellow temperament
he'd be pummeled to pulp back on mainland fo sho
    if dope got out Bad Dog's a pooh bear

Bellows that rumble, paws big as my head
    lord of gang realm, he'd cram you with lead
yet naked sans knife, brash respite from fear
    steels balls for a taste of tentative cheer

Splayed in palm shade, cuffs in surf flung
    gentle mirth tumbles from bile-stung tongue
softens creased face so long hate-hurt steeped
    ventures a smile that makes lava rock weep

---

urban dictionary: "braddah" = brother, "fo sho" = for sure

Phoenix

If I jam my mind with a thousand puzzles
    I almost drown out the doubt
If I cut deep, might blank out the blows
    crowd out the rage in your shout

If I cram my day so I nearly collapse
    I don't see your scowl of disdain
nor hear sneer that wilts exclamation to stammer
    I am through with your venomous shame

I will not clutter my soul with forgiveness
        no longer stifle the fury
nor cloak the ache with relentless regret
        I shan't bear the cross of your misery

I will still the din, the quivering heart
        and savor a ramble through thorns
laugh loud for the girl whose smile you smothered
 splendid duckling, I shall not swan

Stay

I cringe when I sense your shame at my pain
you flame red chagrined and shush me still
I swallow my cries and hide my shame

My fingers are frozen, my toes are aflame
can't quiet the tingling in numb withered limbs
not sure you could even imagine my pain

Enthralling chemo, savior and bane
each moment alive attests to sheer will
I stifle my cries and embrace my shame

As fluorescent days dim I am almost insane
crave your smell and your arms and your hope yet still
I don't know that I want you to share my pain

Ache knows no sleep, on my dreams stakes dread claim
I lose most of dinner, can't keep down this swill
pardon my wails, it's just such a shame

Crank up the morphine, sweet damning refrain
don't push me away, we will conquer this hill
I know it kills you to see me in pain
Don't you dare cry. I am not ashamed.

Brian Cromwell

Another Day In Eternity

The mummy of Irethorrou (500 BCE, Akhim, Egypt), on display at the
California Palace of the Legion of Honor, San Francisco

At night, once the visitors and docents have all left,
darkness surrounds Irethorrou like gauze,

and he can rest. He checks to see if his heart, viscera, and name
are still in the canopic jars near his sarcophagus. They are.

The silence of ancient resin, myrrh, cinnamon, and sawdust
pulses, the certainty of eternity in the preservation of the physical.

He tries but can't quite remember the seventy days of natron, dessicating
his skin so it would not decompose, the satisfaction of forever.

Now, his *ka*, resting inside himself, can receive nourishment,
shadow's substance, a sigh without the need for breath.

Now, his human-headed bird *ba* whistles, begins another night exploring
the museum, the Impressionists of Paris, Japanese prints, Rodin.

Outside, fog-draped pines and cypress endure the night;
the golf course's dark, damp fairways and greens relax.

At dawn's first dab lighting dark sky, Irethorrou, his *ka* and *ba*
together again, re-poses for another day in eternity.

Nostalgia

A Lionel train makes the same stop
at the same station, under a cracking sign.

A faded schedule hugs the ticket window,
an unswept stub on the floor.

The caboose leaves, clears the bend,
disappears into the plastic mountain tunnel.

Tracks ache under whirring wheels
that cannot say good-bye.

I cannot find my tickets, but those painted trees,
aren't they just as beautiful as ever?

Rebecca Ashcraft

Lullaby

Numerous research studies assert that nurses who routinely work nights are at higher risk than the general population for developing various cancers, cardiovascular conditions, gastrointestinal disorders, reproductive problems, depression, alterations in metabolism, and dysfunctional relationships. To that list I'd like to add: premature grey hair and really sucky dance moves.

Night differential pay, loosely translated, means "more martinis per debit card," so it makes sense that the young ones sign up. Having recently survived college, many new grads thrive on sleep deprivation and are able to snooze peacefully on needles of heat at midday in sun-soaked rooms. These are our newbies, always willing to pick up overtime—as long as the extra shift doesn't fall on a weekend.

Most older nurses have forgotten why they're here, stuck between the hours of dusk and dawn, in a place that long ago began to feel more like home—than home. During days off, clock numbers have no particular meaning; time away from the hospital means playing computer games past midnight, scrubbing windowsills at 3:00 AM, and dozing off at sunrise in the middle of a bad murder mystery. These are our dinosaurs, consistently rigid with scheduled lunch breaks—even in the midst of a crisis.

My own experience on nights began, as many epic adventures do, as a little test. I had only intended to *peek* over the top of that windswept bluff, stumbled a little on the ledge, then managed to lose my footing completely. I spent the next eighteen years in a slow-motion slide down the face of Night Shift Cliff. It was a rocky incline lacking those random trees that jut out of the hillsides in cartoons.

My first nursing job, at the Phoenix Indian Medical Center, required I work days, evenings, and nights. I did not yet have children, so I was unfamiliar with the concept of staying up all night sober. My initial foray into night shift, often referred to as "crossing over to the dark side," was not a success by anyone's standards, especially those of Mary, my nursing supervisor. I cried for no reason. I threw up. I got nauseated and *couldn't* throw up. I laughed uncontrollably one morning as the sun rose because—well—there we were, all just sitting at the nurses' station, and our patients were sleeping, and our charts were on the desk, and we had our *pens* and were all wearing white, and—you know—the coffee cups were there and stuff, and it was just freaking *hilarious*. Imagine my disappointment when I realized I didn't need all that beer in college to have fun. I just had to sit up all night and wait for the endorphins to kick in. Shoot! I'd have saved tons of cash.

The end of my mandatory night shift assignments came after a particularly memorable loss in my perpetual battle with slumber. I'd barely managed to stay awake between hourly rounds, and at 4:00 AM I walked robotically into a four-bed ward at the end of the hall. Three ladies scheduled for surgery later that morning were deep in sleep, and as I shined my flashlight on each one I became a little drowsier. I aimed the light at the fourth bed. Empty.

Hmmm.

That bed had been empty all night, but it hadn't looked quite so *empty* on my earlier rounds. My eyelids tried to lift for a better glimpse. I salivated. I turned the flashlight off.

It seemed like a stellar idea at the time to lay *just* my head on the mattress. Wow. It felt great. So, naturally, I thought I'd ease just my shoulders onto the bed—in spite of the awkwardly uncomfortable angle—and I was right! That felt simply marvelous, too.

Needless to say, it turned out to be a pretty *bad* idea because, while I didn't lose my actual job over that decision, I did lose at least two years of projected life expectancy when I woke with a snore—curled on the bed in full sunlight with my stethoscope sprawled at my feet. Three middle-aged, totally expressionless Navaho women watched from their beds as I—their young nurse in the new, white dress—drooled on the back of my hand.

I worked a few years in daylight and was once again faced with shift dilemma after my daughter, Abi, was born. When she slept at longer intervals, I realized I'd be home for her waking hours if I went ahead—bit the bullet—and worked nights.

It was not an easy transition. At home I could squeeze in a *little* sleep during the all-night Baby Rodeo; not so in the Intensive Care Unit, even if the census was low. One night I sat wrapped in a blanket, head bobbing on my springy neck, and asked a coworker who worked six nights a week how she did it. I'll never forget her face. Framed in hair she'd cut herself (she and her hippie husband had four children and lived in fear of appearing extravagant), her eyes bugged out and bored through to the essence of my very being as she whispered, "When you know you *have* to do it, it doesn't seem so bad. Once you *don't* have to do it, it becomes intolerable." Yeesh. That memory still creeps me out.

Twenty-five years of moving between states, changing hospitals within cities, and working for nursing agencies have exposed me to lots of other nocto-moms. A nurse in Kansas City with three young children explained one Sunday morning, as she hurried past me to retrieve her coat from the locker room, why she wouldn't work any other shift. Wrapping a scarf around her neck, she said she'd zip by the grocery store after church so she could bake lemon bars for a potluck later that day and cupcakes for her daughter's birthday the next. She pulled on gloves, hat, and boots as she explained how she would sleep for a couple of hours after the potluck and see me back at work that night. (And, yes—she would deliver the cupcakes, along with some Pink Power Ranger napkins she'd buy on the way to her daughter's school, the next morning before noon.) Her words stayed with me: "I can easily do what I need to on very little sleep, and I can sleep all I want when they're done growing up."

Here's a little rant on one of my peeviest pet peeves: Night shift workers do not take "naps" after work. When they sleep during the day, they are Sleeping During The Day. Most "normal" people seem to believe that because the sun is out, it can't be real sleep. For example, let's say I had a chance to sleep eight hours—perhaps I got home just as Abi left for school and was sleeping soundly by the time she got to home room, or maybe she had play practice after school, so my alarm was set to ring later than usual. The phone calls invariably came, and even if the caller knew my schedule by heart, the voice that woke me was practically choked with surprise. "Oh, you're *napping*? It's two o'clock!" Here's a simple calculation that comes automatically with enough practice: Two o'clock in the afternoon equals two o'clock in the morning for "normal" people. Simple, right?

I slept with the ringer on in case the school needed to get in touch with me. They called exactly once in those eighteen years (the only time the ringer was off—more on that later), but I got plenty of calls inquiring about whether I needed lawn service, broader cell phone coverage, or more frequent newspaper delivery. I never put one of those obnoxious signs by the doorbell that said, "Shhhh! Day Sleeper!" for fear that someone might break in and kill me in my sleep for leaving such an obnoxious sign. Therefore, I also had face-to-face meetings with people inquiring about my potential need for lawn work, phone service, and newspapers.

I took full responsibility for my decision to work nights, so I tried not to complain (too much) about neighbors who waited until they saw me drag my deflated carcass through the front door before simultaneously starting their lawnmowers, hedge trimmers, and snow blowers, while ordering their children and/or injured dogs to play under my bedroom window. Earplugs, eye covers, white noise machines, dreams of Neighbor Revenge—God invented them all for a reason.

Night nurses' lives are particularly obstacle-laden when children are too young for school, or school is not in session due to weekends, summers, holidays, snow days, heat days, "teacher workshops" (my favorite ruse), or illness of the children themselves. Luckily, we night nurses have taken care of sick people in the dark for so long that we can easily take care of sick people in the light with our eyes closed. But children who are well—and *ecstatic* about the bomb-threat school cancellation—do not usually "get" the please-let-Mama-sleep-for-two-hours message.

Early experimentation with day sleep when Abi was not yet two proved disastrous. My great plan was to come home after work, stay up until she took her morning nap, then lie down with her until—what—was I thinking she'd take an eight-hour nap? I'm still not sure where that was headed, but here's the way that first morning went: I arrived home in one piece as planned. After feeding her breakfast, I took Abi into my bedroom and shut the door so she wouldn't even dream of wandering around the house. I sprinkled alphabet blocks around her on the floor and—here's the scary part—for some insane reason, I decided to sit on the bed to watch her play. Did I not have any memory of my Near Bed Experience at the Indian hospital? Anyway, there I was— watching her stack blocks and checking her eyes with each blink for signs of impending sleepiness.

I, myself, blinked extra hard once and when I opened my eyes I found an entire alphabet village built at my feet—and no Abi. Yes, the bedroom door was wide open, which could only mean some cell-phone-coverage representative had broken in and invited her to go on a few sales calls. I ran down the stairs three at a time, heart beating too wildly to let my brain think about breathing. I rounded the corner by the dining room and there she was—sprawled on the kitchen counter wearing only her diaper, scooping huge globs from the butter dish into her mouth. When she saw me, she smiled and raised her yellow hand in a Squinty-Buddha-High-Cholesterol salute. Unfortunately, my lungs found enough air for a scream at that moment and ruined the good time for both of us. After that, Grandma offered to keep her during my "naps."

When Abi was old enough to understand the occasional need to play quietly while I slept for a couple of hours, I still awoke more than once to a very scary sight: my adorable daughter's face less than an inch from mine, resting on the bed, watching me sleep. I think it was the warm gusting of air from her tiny nostrils on my eyelids that did it, but my heart lodged in my throat as I struggled not to get angry—after all, she was playing quietly and hadn't tried to wake me up. She'd smile and say, "Mama! You're awake!" What could I do? I'd get up and remind myself that an hour of sleep is better than no sleep at all. (I believe Mother Theresa put that exact quote on a bumper sticker.)

A coworker in St. Louis told me her husband was in charge of watching their four boys while she slept one day, and when she woke up they all had new B-B guns. Including her husband. She tried to kill him with her bare hands, but ran out of time when she needed to hop in the shower and go back to work.

Another nurse at a hospital in Anchorage said her husband forgot to feed the kids one day and quickly let them eat whatever they wanted when he heard his wife stirring. She had a stick protruding from the back of her hair and when I pointed it out during shift report, she said, "Oh, that's where that went. Jacob had a fit in the back seat when they dropped me off tonight because he couldn't find his sucker after he threw it at his sister."

When Abi started kindergarten I had to adapt to a new schedule. The days of driving around until she fell asleep in her car seat, then pulling into a grocery store parking lot to snooze alongside her, were officially over. All those allegedly well-meaning shoppers who tapped tentatively on the driver's window to make sure we were still alive would just have to find some other goody-two-shoes activity to fill their days! (In my defense, Abi woke up if I tried to carry her into the house and grocery stores just felt so safe to me. We all know criminals don't eat real food.)

Kindergarten only happened in the mornings, so I'd rush home to be asleep by 8:00 AM, wake with the alarm at 11:00, and be in line with the other parents by 11:30. The school required that parents come into the building, but not into the class-room, so we stood against a glass wall by the principal's office where we could see the kids as they approached down a long hallway. Every day their teacher admonished her uncoordinated pupils to stay single file, don't run, don't touch, don't hit, slow down, etc.—until Abi eventually broke from the pack, ran toward me lightning fast and jumped into my outstretched arms from about five feet away.

I had horrible visions of us crashing through the glass and onto the principal's lap, so I stood with my left leg braced against the wall, right leg lunged in front of me, and heart about to burst with joy that she could possibly be so happy to see me. I know she recognized me from afar thanks to the same jeans-tee-shirt-sandal combi-nation I wore every single day, and I still feel lucky that she never once veered off course into the arms of a mom wearing printed cotton capris with a matching sweater set. Or perhaps Abi was drawn to the Mystery Hospital Smell, which those brightly checkered moms did not emit.

On a day that I must have looked exceptionally tired, a kind friend suggested I sleep longer than three hours the next day. "Don't set your alarm," he said, "I'll get Abi and take her to lunch; you can call whenever you wake up." Wow. A whole day! (Spoiler alert: This was the day I got my only phone call from the school.) The kind friend apparently got caught up in the generosity of the moment and completely forgot about having a job. While at work the next day, he completely forgot about my extra-long "nap." I woke up (disappointingly close to noon anyway) to an answering machine tape full of snide messages from the school nurse, demanding to know if I "felt like picking up" my daughter that day. I dialed the school and made sure I wasn't on speakerphone before asking why the angry nurse didn't call any contacts in Abi's file. She had some lame response about it not being her job. Intelligence not being my strong suit under stress, I came back with an even lamer response about nurses in general and hung up. When I picked Abi up and asked what happened in the nurse's office, she said, "Oh, it was fun! She let me stay and watch her eat her lunch." Abi is one person who will not have those awkward silences when she starts seeing a therapist.

There were a few more glitches in Operation Abi over the years. I slept fifteen minutes into a tennis practice, twenty minutes into a voice lesson, and almost forgot completely about inventing games for the sixth grade Valentine's Day party (I must have been sound asleep when I volunteered for that job). Luckily, my merry band of sleep-deprived mothers helped me out at work the night before, and the party was a smashingly hyperactive success.

The worst glitch of all, in terms of public embarrassment, came during a volley-ball game that I screwed up by agreeing to act as line judge on a day I'd had no sleep. After what seemed like several hours of play, the echoing gymnasium noises ceased abruptly and I glanced up at the referee, standing on his perch at the net and asking for my ruling. "In or out?" he demanded.

Okay, here's the deal: I'd been drifting in my usual Daytime Underwater Haze (DUH), staring at the knee socks of a girl from the opposing team who was serving to my right, and wishing our girls had those socks, only in our colors, and without the little fuzzy hippo face, or whatever their school animal was, when a ball apparently hit somewhere near the line to my left. I stared back at the referee, swallowed hard, and tentatively pointed my arms down to signal "in." The boos were deafening—from fans of both teams. The ball was clearly "out" to those who were watching. Why didn't the referee just take a vote, for gosh sakes?

A few years ago I found myself in a situation involving a young coworker who had a ten-month-old daughter at home. Sometime after midnight her patient crashed, and several of us were helping in the room when the young nurse's frustrated husband called. He couldn't get their baby to stop crying and knew she needed her mother to sing a special lullaby that always worked. Luckily, this nurse was good at her job and multi-tasked in a way for which her generation is famous. With the phone cradled between her left ear and shoulder, singing so softly we couldn't hear her over the chaos in the room, she ran the crash cart drug drawer—popping ends off epi and atropine syringes, handing them off in the right order, mixing pressors, spiking saline bags, etc. I was so impressed.

That scenario returns to me often, and pierces my heart every single time. It's very likely the same bit of pain felt by the man who begs for fortune cookies at the gas station after forgetting about his son's "International Day" at school, or by the woman who extracts a small, sticky, Hello Kitty notebook from her briefcase during a business presentation.

One day I'll get Abi's perspective on all those dinners I rushed through so I could get to work on time. I'll hear how sad she was when she wanted to cuddle on the couch, but I had to leave; how happy she was when I came home with a red-and-white striped bag from the hospital gift shop with the newest silly candy—a mailbox of edible letters, or band-aid bubble gum.

But that will be her story. I can only speak for those of us sandwiched between the newbies and the dinosaurs—not there for the extra party money or a break from hours of solitaire. We were there because we didn't want to miss a basketball game. Our daughters had dance recitals and, by God, we would bring the cookies. Our sons needed rides to swim practice every single day of the summer, and sleeping in the car under a big shady tree is almost as restful as being in bed at home.

If someone pointed out our crazy behavior, attempted to explain the benefits of sleeping at night like "normal" people, the message was lost. For there were certain moments—like the privilege of watching a daughter walk nervously to a piano bench in front of a hundred people, or the honor of waving back at a son who was sent to play outfield—that assured us we were on the right path.

Those moments turned my slippery trip down that cliff into one thrilling ride.

Charlotte Melleno

White Shoulders

My mother's perfume is bottled in a round
glass coffin, sits on a shelf reserved—
this is the scent she touched to her throat
before the blue whale swallowed
her body.

When my mother woke at dawn her eyes
were green, darkened as she staggered
through her day. Nothing went
as she wished, couldn't convey the difference
between rose and thorn—
some afternoons so black with blue
her sobs threatened to carry us
all away. Our apartment
might well have been
Dresden, bombers buzzing low over
the kitchen sink while she ducked
washing dishes, cautioned me to
wipe them dry or else
we'd be incinerated.

This is an ode to loss. A rough nod
to an early death, shocking in simplicity—
a heart attack on Wednesday—they thought
she'd make it but she battled my father
for scissors, begged him—
cut the ties around my wrists.
He did and left when
the nurses tied her up again.
She died fighting her heart.

After, I'd walk around Stow Lake
huffing the heavy air, found enough silence
for a conversation, but she wasn't there.
Not then, not for many years and when she came—
as a small girl in a plaid hat, fragrant
with her scent—I knew her
and she held my hand.

Everything I Know Is True

after Naomi Shihab Nye

You are accessible in the way
that water is
when you turn the faucet, knowing
it will flow out.
I am that certain about you.
I don't need to crane my brain
around your poems, small
seashells of sound
holding the entire ocean.
Everything I know is true
about myself—the wrinkles on top
of my hands, how my hair wilts
and wires in muggy weather,
my self-centeredness, the deep well
of abandonment I fell into
as a child
and will never rise above
although I *fight*—
you say pajamas and I feel redeemed.
The truest, softest things are
in your voice
like a receiving blanket or the fur
collar of her coat
the day she hugged and left me
to grow up alone.

The Virgin Mary Goes Line Dancing

Doesn't she ever get tired of holding
the frail, comforting the sick-at-heart
or body? Is she ever sick
of being a haloed, blue-robed caretaker—
Star of the Sea, Mother of the Universe—
and does she ever want to crawl
under flowered flannel blankets,
have God bring her a cup
of lavender tea or give her a manicure?

Would the rule hold up in heaven:
What happens in Vegas stays in Vegas
if she took time off to play
the slots or hunger after a Chippendale dancer?
Would she frown like a nun
in a long black gown but travel the Appalachian Trail
in secret to stuff a few bucks
down the waistband of his hot pants, marvel
at his wonders?

I find her in the ladies room
of a Country-Western bar one Friday night,
her green cowboy boots embroidered
with Christmas trees. Weeping, she yearns
to be like others but remains herself—
timeless, somewhere
between seventeen and two-thousand-and-ten.
My questions fall like dominoes
in a nursing home.
She asks, "Want a hug?"
"You're incorrigible," I respond.
She nods her head and God glides in,
blows away her tears with a cloudy mouth
and takes her home at last call.

Lisa Kerr

The Girl Who Grew Herself Up as a Bird, Norway 1349

She was the only human
> found alive in the mountain valley
>> town of Jostedalen after the scourge.

She toddled out into view, accidentally,
> a timid child-grouse searching the dust hungrily
>> for leaves and insects. Her feathers,

hot tufts of brown and gray,
> plumed and drifted around her.
>> A human child molting.

She darted away to escape eyes, hands, stunned-open
> mouths approaching at human speed.
>> She had been free

of all work but survival, of sibling hands petting
> and slapping, of language—
>> the pressure to achieve vowels, syllables.

One of our women went to her alone, hands extended
> to welcome her back to the land of our living.
>> When she found the child's waist,

lifted her squirming to the hip, every bird
> in that valley took wing all at once, infected the sky
>> like a plague of memory and forgetting.

Wild Rabbits in San Rafael

The rabbits have come on long, bent legs
to see what I'm about on this bench
under the trees. They will be disappointed
to find me sitting unproductive,
guessing the names of unfamiliar things.
At home, I know the wrens and buntings,
pine and oleander, yellow foxes who roam
at dusk. Here, I am eager to learn
what to call each foreign tree and flower,
how to lure the local creatures to rest
by my feet. And for a moment, watching rabbits,
I forget about the things in my body
no one has named yet. About how waiting
for a name, an answer, a diagnosis
is like wandering in a strange forest,
praying the animals and plants
who rule there have secrets, charms
and will be generous.

Deer among Rabbits

This morning as I walked in San Rafael,
I found myself across the fence
from a gathering of deer and rabbits.
They were among high grasses and clover
in the small yard of a Dominican Sisters' home.
What was I to them? They hardly took notice.
While I, enraptured, fell down
in thanks, my fingers in the fence wire,
knees bleeding into stone.

Louis B. Jones

Empathy and Characterization

I've heard that Flannery O'Conner, somewhere in her fiction, has a pretty accurate portrait of life on an army base; however, it seems to have been the case that she'd never set foot inside an army base; and once, when she was asked how she got the details so right without having had the first-hand experience herself, she answered that she'd one time ridden past the front gate of an army base; and that was enough; the glimpse of the buildings beyond the gates permitted her to make a whole world of surmises about what life was like inside those gates. She was able to see what was important in there. Maybe it was only something as simple as a ring of stones that had been set with care around a central flagpole. Or just the building-standards' utilitarian simplicity. She could see what a logical, if peculiar, society it was. That wedge-shaped glimpse through a gate allowed her to construct a world, and over time, an army base grew inside her.

There's a poem by Emily Dickinson that gets at the same kind of sovereignty of the intuitive mind over mere facts' corroboration. It's a short poem on the subject of how limited Miss Dickinson's existence seems to have been. The first stanza goes like this:

> I never saw a Moor—
> I never saw the Sea—
> Yet I know how the Heather looks
> And what a Billow be.

"The sea" of course will be seen as a metaphor for the physical aspect of love—sex—or in this case, about not getting any. The modern reader, debauched as he is in Freud, will even see a masturbatory wish in the conjured wave, which the poet herself might or might not. Her words have a literal meaning, too, which I believe she must have intended. She seems to believe that she really doesn't have to make the trip to the seashore, let alone wade in waist-deep. She seems to contend that her mental picture of a wave, as furnished by literature and art and other second-hand experience, combined perhaps with a little splashing in the bathtub in her Amherst home, will provide her with all she needs to know about waves. In other words, this world of ours has been a "virtual" world since long before the 3-D computer-interface came along. Miss Dickinson's further implication is that plenty of people who may have had the privilege of playing at the seashore for days, might yet have a relatively dim idea of what a wave is. They might have not noticed much about a wave, especially if they haven't been paying the kind of close attention a poet pays. I'm sure she's right about that.

I personally have never seen the Parthenon. And I probably never will. As things are lining up in my life, lately, it looks like any project of "Seeing the Parthenon" will be quietly moving over to the list of things I never got around to in life—along with skydiving, hiking in the Dolomites, giving Joyce's *Ulysses* a second and closer reading—the list of pleasures we'll call our lives complete without having gotten to.

I could tell you a lot about the Parthenon. I was a Classics major at school, and I could make a bore of myself, on the topic of the whole Acropolis, and everything the Acropolis means about Periclean Athens and the course of Western Civilization, or how those buildings forecast the shape of our individual souls today. Plenty of people have never seen the Parthenon, or the Acropolis, but they are all people whose lives were formed by the ideals those buildings announced. My point, of course, is that I don't need to go to Athens. Emily Dickinson's "seashore" is my Parthenon. I've already benefited from the Parthenon so profoundly, exploring it and assimilating it to myself—my life has been so well fed on the Parthenon—that the actual sight of it might disappoint me. Maybe the actual Parthenon, if I come one day to stand before it, will seem small, or will seem to need hosing off. The same goes for Walden Pond, by the way. Anybody who has read Thoreau's electrifying book doesn't need to go to Massachusetts and get off Highway 129 to look at it. I have just now this morning Google-Earthed "Walden Pond," and I can see from the aerial satellite view, as I descend through the blizzard of pixels, that the easiest way to take in the pond nowadays would be to pull off at the Dunkin' Donuts that today stands directly across the highway from the shore.

So my general plan, in speaking today to my writing friends, is an encomium to the imaginary life, especially a life lived according to the rule of empathy. In those hours you spend at your work table, dreaming up things that never were, you are doing something as important in society as, say, the work of a doctor or an engineer, comparatively speaking. Let me follow this useful comparison. If a person is unwell and needs the right medicine to be prescribed—or if a person wants to cross from Marin to San Francisco and needs a dependable bridge—well, in those cases a competent doctor or engineer is called for. But a writer's job in society is almost prior to—and antecedent to—a doctors' or an engineers', because a writer, if the writing is good, will be providing us with our dreams. And providing us with our assumptions. Even engineers need their dreams and assumptions, and doctors too. A writer can furnish us with reasons for crossing that bridge; or, I dare say, reasons for seeking the medicine and preserving health and life. Consider the three or four books in your own life that shed a useful light on your existence. Those books—even if you've grown since then, and left them behind—were at least as important as certain bridges you may have crossed once.

Now, everything I'm saying pertains if, as a writer, you're good at your work. And when you're at your workbench, the one superpower you are equipped with is empathy. It's your power of empathy that will keep lifting you to new views, and new situations, your power of empathy that will keep rescuing and surprising – surprising even you, as author. (Incidentally, all this seems to be as true in real life as in the pages of literature.) Empathy will be your flashlight and your stethoscope and your Swiss Army knife, empathy your prying-bar and your can-opener, empathy your magic decoder ring. In the invention of fictional characters, you're making virtual people who will have consequences in the real world. The world has been changed and impressed by Shakespeare's Shylock and Homer's Achilles, Harriet Beecher Stowe's Uncle Tom, and (more contemporaneously) Michael Chabon's young bisexual Jewish men, and Amy Tan's Chinese-American woman. A writer's real medium—I hope this is already an axiom among us—a writer's real medium is characterization. Plot, language, theme, all those other elements are subordinated to the iron caprice of the cranky little personalities set loose in the text. And the great characters—the Othello or the Leopold Bloom, or Anna Karenina's husband Alexei, or Emma Bovary or Septimus Smith—can be delivered only in the quiet, solitary theatre of the author's empathy.

So how shall we love our characters? How are we to love them as the Lord loves his creatures?

The question goes back to the mystery of what your novel is "About." That is, not merely its plot—not that kind of "aboutness"—but your novel's reason for being, the initial cramp it was born from. Every book has its own innate, incalculable "x" factor. Nabokov used to say of human nature that a personality is formed partly by genes, partly by environment, and largely by the "mysterious x factor." Your novel, like a human being, is going to thrive according to its own quirky, secret rules of valuation and perception. I think if you were trying to track down the physiology of this "x" factor in a work of fiction—this halo, or this perfume, this pheromone—one place to look would be in your story's Narrative Tone. "Narrative Tone" is a concept you'll find discussed in any number of how-to-write-a-novel manuals, a concept up there with plot and theme and diction and dialogue, et cetera, as one of the compositional elements that comprise a work's total artistic strategy. It's just your own natural way of saying things—whether you like to use big words or little, long sentences or short, specific details or big abstractions, argumentative force or disinterested analysis, abrupt zigzagging or smooth transitions. Your own Narrative Tone is something that comes totally naturally and unself-consciously to you. It's not to be scrutinized or messed with. But it acts as the spectacles—or stereopticon or viewfinder—for the reader to see and experience events, and it crucially establishes the reader's emotional distance from the events of the story: some kinds of narration permit no space to intervene between reader and story, no space of irony or humor or skepticism: so they require us to care deeply about the characters—for example, Tillie Olsen's "I Stand Here Ironing"—and never see the character's concerns as trivial or absurd or funny. Other stories allow us to stand off at a little distance: their narrative tone licenses us to be amused by the characters' tribulations—for instance Jane Austen's unmarried girls. In a novel I've been reading this month, Muriel Sparks's "Memento Mori," the approach of death, one-by-one, to a whole social group of sweet, elderly, slightly senile Londoners is actually rendered as amusing. In one scene, a sweet old lady is dispatched when she is beaten to death by a burglar, and Ms. Spark manages to make the two-sentence anecdote of her murder almost comical, like a sort of pratfall.

Jane Austen, in her own way, invites us to stand back and be amused and slightly judgmental. Her *Pride and Prejudice* begins, "It is a truth universally acknowledged, that a single man in possession of a good fortune, must be in want of a wife." That unmistakable sarcasm licenses us to take her characters more lightly. By contrast, Amy Tan's *Bonesetter's Daughter* begins "These are the things I know are true," in its tone a signal that what we're about to read isn't funny.

So Narrative Tone will indicate how gravely or how lightly we are to take characters' problems. Tone establishes an "empathic distance."

So let's move beyond this, and deeper. Narrative Tone, along with reader-empathy, depends in turn partly on the author's conception of how "realistic" the characters and the story are supposed to be. Some writers give us *realistic* people and situations—Hemingway, Updike, Jonathan Franzen, Joyce Carol Oates, J.D. Salinger. Other writers give us patently contrived people, who in real life would appear as grotesques or cartoons—Charles Dickens's Londoners with all their tics and obsessions, Franz Kafka's nightmare situations. Let us say that there's a scale, or spectrum: at one end is "Artifice," where the events of the story are improbable and contrived; at this end of the spectrum lives "magic realism" and Franz Kafka, and Milton's *Paradise*

Lost. The other end of the spectrum is "mimesis"—that is, the attempt at portraying or imitating realistic, naturalistic events; at this end of the spectrum is Hemingway, say. Most writers lie somewhere in between—like Flannery O'Connor or Jane Austen; their characters are not exactly "grotesques" or "caricatures," but their noses have been lengthened slightly, their voices sharpened, their tics exaggerated. We suspend disbelief in reading of their foibles, all the while taking pleasure in their artificiality, that is, in the artifice itself. The artifact itself. The *art* of Jane Austen and Flannery O'Connor. We're taking pleasure in the fine minds of their authors. We "empathize" with those characters only to the degree that the author has licensed us.

So, I think, or hope, I've been getting into the nuts-and-bolts of the "empathy" phenomenon, and hope to go a step further now.

These issues of Narrative Tone and, deeper in, artificiality of characterization, depend on a certain basic element of the story which is built into its genes at its conception. Or (here's a metaphor just barely worth going for) this is an element of story which is built into the quantum at the Big-Bang moment of the birth of the universe in which a given story has its life. I'm talking about the story's "Aboutness" again, an "Aboutness" more pervasive to the story than any plot-summary could express, but which is connected with plot. Every story is "About" something. Every plot has as its seed a certain problem: some kind of problem: something in the world is incorrect. There's been an adultery, or just a flirtation or a temptation. Or a cancer has metastasized. Or there's been a murder, or a theft. Or a lie was told. Or a war has been declared. Or an insult was inflicted. Or society enshrines a prejudice. A story is built around some kind of defect in the world. If the world had no defects, then there would be no story. (If the world indeed had no defects, we'd still be in the Garden of Eden, and have no need of prisons or churches or schools. Nor any need of this "narrative art" either, with its own peculiar offer of redemption.)

In the course of any fictional story, the defect which the author has identified is either ironed out or not. In other words, it's the writer's job to first spot out some kind of manifest "evil," implicit in Creation. Now some books' notion of evil is just for kids. In Ian Fleming's 007 novels, the nemesis is a shady maleficent empire called SMERSH. In other books, maybe it's Adolph Hitler or Darth Vader. Maybe it's a scheming, seducing woman. Maybe it's "Capitalism" that is the manifest evil of the world, as in the fictions of certain early twentieth-century novelists in the days when the literati were all lefties. Much of E.L. Doctorow's early writing depends on our seeing capitalism as the original force of discord in Creation: it menaces the good folks, and it's what corrupted the bad guys. In similar other modern writing, the defect in the world is some abstract social ill, like homophobia, or sexism or racism. But really, what's immediately and directly at stake is never any abstract -ism. It's always the sovereign character. If there's a Nazi, he *chose* Nazism. Nazism didn't come out from its deep cave and choose him. If there's racism at work in a story, then individual human souls, in their frailty, made the choice of racism. The less sophisticated reader likes to hear stories in which the "evil" lies outside ourselves, in anti-semitism or capitalism, or Nazis, or in wild Indians. Something *not* us. After all, listening to a well-told story is a primitive pleasure, a pleasure that began around the campfire, and the rapt audience has always loved the shiver of hearing the twig-snap in the dark *outside* the circle of light. Part of what storytelling does is it defines our circle of light. We like that. We like to hear of fiends and monsters, and then their eradication.

But certain readers go to fiction not as a temporary escape from the world, but to get a closer knowledge of the world. Some fiction is really aimed at the grown-up in us. It's why some of the best fiction is boring and difficult—take Proust or James or Joyce as instances—while some of the worst fiction is instantly lovable. The less sophisticated reader can find it hard to empathize with characters he doesn't "identify with." To "identify with" a Captain Ahab or an Alexei Karenin or a Kate Croy, the effort requires the unfamiliar mental pain of holding two opposed ideas in the mind simultaneously. For some of us, that's like having the on/off switch turned *simultaneously* "on" and "off." It asks us to see some evil in the good characters, some good in the evil characters, and indeed as readers to practice actual empathy.

So different novelists will identify the "defect" in Creation in their own ways. Maybe you're Jane Austen and your world is "All About" the terrible equation of marriage and prostitution—the necessity in English bourgeois society for a young woman to catch a rich man. Well, that's a serious undertaking for a writer, and Miss Austen used the most exquisite tones of irony to paint that picture. Austen's novels are, largely, about discernment of character traits; the suspense in them arises from whether true virtue will ever be discerned in a world of specious ignoble successes; the question in Jane Austen is always whether the one who has patience and integrity will be picked out from among the flashier types.

Or maybe you're Dostoevsky and what's at stake in your world is a frankly religious problem, the moral and spiritual redemption of the soul. Or maybe you're Raymond Carver and, as instanced in his portraits of drunks and liars, it's human incontinence and weakness. Or you're John Steinbeck, author of *The Grapes of Wrath*, and the manifest "evil" in the world is a systemic social and political unfairness besetting the common man in the class system.

So you see, as a novelist inventing a world, how you define this "evil" that was seeded in the Garden of Eden will determine the moral force-of-gravity on your particular planet. Things do feel a good deal heavier on Dostoevsky's planet than they do on Jane Austen's. Or, say, on P.G. Wodehouse's planet, where things are so light they're helium-filled.

Lately I've been admiring Henry James for his understanding of "evil." Of course as a commonly used word, "evil" isn't so much a useful or clear predicate as just a vague vituperation, mostly dangerous and hurtful. But James seems to get at a realistic portrait of what actual intentional "evil" may be. He seems to see the real thing, moving in the world, in people's hearts and in people's drawing-rooms, and in their marriages and families. The novel "Washington Square" is a scary portrait of a father-daughter relationship, in which a father—a popular, powerful, charming man of great prestige—systematically destroys the self-esteem of his daughter, as well as all her life chances. The daughter is a little overweight and awkward, and he demolishes her by erosion over the years, through the power of his charming sarcastic wit. Apparently he does this for his own aggrandizement, habitually, and of course for the beautiful exercise of wit itself. And in "Portrait of a Lady" the scheming of Gilbert Osmond and Madame Merle around the fate of an innocent young woman— and in "Wings of the Dove" the pair of young lovers who plot to break the heart and steal the fortune of a terminally ill young woman— in all these instances James sets his stethoscope directly on a few rather realistic monsters, without flinching. Those people could be *us*. James's peculiarly clinical artistic insight was into the sick complicity of the victim; and the pragmatic rationality of the vicious; and with a coroner's touch, he practiced an empathy that seems disinterested to the point of being angelic. I almost think he must have been a cold-blooded man himself. I've never read a biography of James, so I don't know. He may have been an unhappy man, at least.

So now I'm coming almost to the end of all I have to say about this phenomenon of empathy in fiction. It may be clear, my personal feeling is that empathy is what can save us. One does wish there were more empathy in the world, and it seems that fiction is where we rehearse redemption, what there may be of it.

When you're at your table working over a manuscript, you have a very important chance to get outside yourself. During most of our daylight hours, we operate on the assumption that we are separate, finite entities, separate bags of skin, containing separate sovereign consciousnesses, limited in time and space. This shared assumption provides a basis of society. The real-estate-like sense of ownership of a "self" for some eighty or so years—as it were, ownership "in fee simple"—is an inescapable category of experience. Like our experience of "time" and our experience of "space," our experience of an autonomous isolated "self" is ineluctable. But when as an artist you create the virtual world of an imaginary human being, you fly beyond the boundaries of yourself and you enter a somewhat *more realistic* realm. The "self" serves a conventional entitlement of participation in a larger, evolving social and cultural organism of morality and wisdom. In that cultural organism, Shylock and Holden Caulfield and Nigger Jim are as consequential as you and I. And the pronoun "I" in that text—that little free-standing Doric column on the page—is a grammatically necessary placeholder: it makes predication possible: it's purely a point-of-view, like a camera-angle.

There's a popular expression that came along in recent years—"Get a life!"— intended as a sort of dismissive insult. It seems to want to convey that *your* concerns are trivial and absurd, and that you ought to take up bigger, more interesting pursuits. In your work as a writer, the world is a place where everybody has already got a life. Everybody without exception has already got a life in full, and is already doing the most important thing, in a theatre of events so vast and so intricately woven that, as artists, we can only represent a few vignettes arbitrarily seized-upon.

In conclusion, let me confess an important doubt and warning. I think the bad news underlying my little sermon is that nothing I've said here will be any help to you when you're back at your work table. You may quickly come to think of everything I've said as forgettable, and even perhaps as airy-fairy or academic, if you like, which it may be. But such news is also bracing, to an artist once freed from the precincts of a writers' conference and driving home alone: such news is invigorating, and a kick-in-the-ass. Everything I've said today will vanish from practical usefulness because, I suppose, nothing can help a working artist. A story's origins lie in an inner world that is incalculable, a world that is infinitely deep and ancient. Likewise, a story's destination in the outer world is incalculable. No one knows where it comes from or where it's going, to do its work. Your only job is to be as unbiased and clear as possible, in the practice of empathy.

Ann Emerson

About Doctor G.

He goes out of his way every time to ask how
I'm doing. He is the tree whispering through

the cracked hospital window, the shiver of white
narcissus, the breeze lifting the skirt of the nurse

opening my door. He is the song in my head that
doesn't stop at night, the way curious medicine

wanders my blood—I no longer go out of my way to
picture the mound of earth dug just my size.

Sometimes someone touches your hand in an
unexpected room and you close your eyes

like the lid of a music box that's been wanting
quiet for years. When I start to die, this is

how it will be: no terrible music, no one taking
my place, his footsteps in silence carrying on.

"About Dr. G." was first published in *Alaska Quarterly Review*, Vol. 28, Nos. 1 & 2 (Spring & Summer), p. 254.

Not the Last

In this story I am an old animal
and not sad in the way people think

about horses vanishing in the West.
Stanford Cancer Center. The hills behind the

research lab are stitched tight with barbed wire.
Things now are just as they said it would be:

steel devices and PKC412.
End-stage: I am a feral horse untouched

by human hands, lithe as grasses on
high plains. Pink gasps of lungs for air.

This isn't the last poem I will write about
orchids on the desks of doctors from grateful

families of the dead. Here, in this closed
room, I grow restless pricked with silver

hooks and tools. I am not sad no one
has figured me out and I do not wonder why things

turn out as they do: my sky pouring gold through
the window, the crack of wind setting me free.

Terri Mason

Untie

These days I live in double knots,
always in two places, one my sister's room,
watching for an ending I don't want to begin.
I take my niece to swimming lessons;
she's in the Turtle group. Sit poolside
while she paddles blinking in the sun,
breathing in sweetness, chlorinated air.

We return to a borrowed house
where the shades are drawn. Turtle goes
to Grandma. I check on the IV,
feed my sister yogurt with live cultures.
She eats all I offer, then vomits in a bin. The nurse
says, at this stage, she can't make use of food.

My stubborn sparring partner is renouncing all
her roles: visual artist, tender mother, struggling
wife. She speaks only word salad so we're learning
a new language, hands and eyes in present tense.

Her skeleton grows eloquent a little more each day,
reveals what I'm afraid, yet curious to know—
What will it take for her to die?
How will it be for me?

When her husband arrives with his guitar,
I go to restaurants, eat burgers, malts, and fries.
It's good to be alive and I will bear the guilt.
Wish I were the type who could flirt up a one night
stand. Awake now to the mysteries in other diners' lives.

Tonight I sleep on a cot at her bedside
in a room we've never shared. Doors I've shut
against her open. Her voice draws me
a picture of the unfamiliar land where
she searches for a car. I have no
compass, just relax and let her drive.

Boundaries

After she dies, I wear my sister's clothes.
We're almost the same size.

For certain tests, I wear a gown.
My confidence leaks out the gaps.

I buy expensive paper, like hers,
take a drawing class.

I scan the edges of my moles—
have they shifted overnight?

Earrings, shawls and skirts are easy to adopt.
I throw away her underwear.

After I am diagnosed, I pack her things away.
Avoid looking in the mirror.

Longing

Had I power to make it so,
my cell phone would be bird
and fly my message straight to
you encoded in a song.

Instead, I stand on a far bank
and watch green rivers flow
carve out cliffs along the
border of what can
and cannot be.

Would I were a cavalier from
long ago, sure my aim was true,
never know haphazard blows,
at least, pretend they were
no more than feathers
less than stones.

Warren Holleman

Group Therapy

A version of this story first appeared as "Girl Talk" in
Pulse: Voices from the Heart of Medicine, November 12, 2010.

I got pregnant. Quit sports, quit school. Quit all my dreams. Brenda looks fit and handsome, despite the scar running down the middle of her face. At six feet tall, she commands respect, even though she speaks in a sweet, high-pitched voice that belies her imposing physique.

We are sitting in a circle: Brenda, six other women, and me. Most are in their thirties and forties, and in their fourth or fifth month of sobriety. They look professional in the suits they assembled from the donations closet.

No one is surprised when Brenda says that, twenty years ago, she trained for the U.S. Olympic volleyball team.

Did you ever compete again? someone asks.

Nope.

Why not?

Brenda shakes her head. The group gives her a moment to think about it, to grieve the loss.

Later, I took up tennis. I was pretty good! Won quite a few tournaments. You know, just local tournaments.

Brenda pauses, then continues. *The people I played with, they were doctors, lawyers, people like that. Which was kinda cool. But this was the eighties, and everybody was using powder cocaine. You know what I mean?*

The older ladies do know what she means. They nod and cast glances around the room.

And something else happened. She took a deep breath. *I met this man.*

Everybody perks up. They are hoping against hope for a good love story. *And you fell in love with him?*

Oh no! I ain't THAT crazy.

Falling in love ain't crazy.

He was seventy years old. I was twenty-five.

Yeah. So why are you telling us about him?

Because I married him.

You what?

Girl. He had money and a four-bedroom house. That sounded soooo good.

Wow!

And that sounded so good.

More nods and smiles and glances. *And?*

And what?

Was it worth it?

Hell no!

Four bedrooms is a lot of real estate.

He was this LITTLE man.

So?

This was his fifth marriage.

I could put up with a lot for four bedrooms.

He was a sick-o.

Girl! What could he do to YOU?

Brenda takes a pregnant pause. She's starting to look angry. *He could beat me. He could belittle me.*

I don't see how.

I was fucked up. Hooked on his money. Hooked on his cocaine.

Brenda looks around the room, then up at the ceiling. She talks to the ceiling: *After I left him, I couldn't afford no more powder. So then I did something REALLY stupid. I got hooked on crack.* She lowers her gaze: *I told you I was fucked up.*

The ladies begin commiserating: *Like WE wasn't fucked up? At least you knew where to come to for help.*

Sure! It only took me fifteen years! She's angry, mostly at herself, but also at the other ladies for trying to cheer her up. *I wasted fifteen years.* Brenda stops talking, but no one dares speak. The only sound is her breathing. She's trying to figure out some way to redeem those fifteen years. Suddenly, she perks up: she's got an idea. *Hey! Maybe you ladies can learn from my mistakes.*

One by one, they respond. *We're listenin. We're learnin. You've helped me see somethin.*

I'm supposed to be leading this group, but so far I haven't said a word. All the ladies appear engaged. Except for Sabrina.

Sabrina is eighteen years old. A few weeks ago she told us she's tired of living on the street. This morning she's been quiet, taking it all in. She's the youngest, the group mascot. Finally, she speaks up.

You said "sick-o"—your husband was a sick-o. What do you mean—sick-o?

He had a lead pipe. He covered it with rubber padding. He just liked to walk around holding it in his hand.

Whoa, says one of the ladies. *Hmm,* says another.

He didn't scare me, 'cause I was a LOT bigger than him.

So what's the problem? Sabrina asks.

He hit me—hard. He put me in a coma. For five days they didn't know if I'd wake up. And what would be left if I did.

Silence.

You do see the scar—right? If ever there was an elephant in the room. It was wide as a pencil and ran from her hairline to halfway down her nose.

Finally, they begin speaking up. *I always wondered how you got that. I was afraid to say anything.* A third lady reaches out to take Brenda's hands: *Oh baby, he hurt you bad.*

That's why I breathe so loud.

You breathe just fine.

I was the type ... Brenda's eyes begin to water. Someone hands her a Kleenex. *I had to learn my lesson the hard way.*

A quiet understanding fills the air. The other women have been there themselves. We let it all sink in.

I'm the one who breaks the silence. *You said you learned your lesson the hard way. From the feeling of the room, I'm sensing that this was a really important lesson, both for you and for all of us.* Nods of recognition around the room. *May I ask what that lesson was?*

Never marry a man for his money—it ain't worth it. If ever it was worth it, it would have been this man. He had a ton of money.

The chorus responds: *I hear you, darlin. You sure got that right. Oh yeah.* Then from the other side of the circle: *Amen. We love you, baby.*

Except for Sabrina, every woman has spoken. All eyes turn to her. *This man, is he still alive?*

Brenda puts her hand on Sabrina's shoulder and leans forward to face her, nearly touching forehead to forehead. *Honey, I don't think he'll EVER die!*

The other women laugh and shake their heads. I relax, thinking that's the end of the session.

But Sabrina has one more thing she'd like to say. *Hey!* Everybody turns in her direction. Sabrina stares Brenda in the eye, but she doesn't say anything.

Brenda breaks the ice: *Yeah?*

Tell me where he is. I'd like that money.

I sure didn't see that coming. It's nine o'clock, time for our break, and I need one.

We're back. I start things off by reminding everybody that this is the last day of the group. The last hour, in fact. All eyes turn to Dorothy.

In all this time, Dorothy has avoided talking about herself, fueling the suspicion that she's hiding something really interesting. I feel tense because Dorothy was assigned to me for individual therapy, and she hasn't opened up with me, either. I tried showing her how to do a family genogram, thinking that something tactile might resonate. She played along, but I could see she wasn't buying it.

Dorothy is a proud woman and, like Brenda, is tall and tough and strong. And, a former athlete—a track and field star. But unlike Brenda, she speaks in a deep, husky, monotone voice.

Five years ago, she says, a bullet sliced her spine in two, leaving her a paraplegic.

The group fires away with questions: how she got shot; how she takes care of herself in that wheelchair; how she drives that big ol' van; how she got the money to pay for the van; how she raised her children. With a wave of her spastic hand, Dorothy dismisses the questions and takes charge.

I've only got one hour. I'm gonna talk about my family genogram.

Everybody sits up in their chairs. We've never heard Dorothy say two sentences in a row.

I came from a dysfunctional family. DYS-functional family. The men went to prison, and the women took care of them. You hear what I'm sayin?

The ladies nod their heads.

Dorothy reaches into her bag and pulls out a sheet of paper. She struggles to unfold it, then lays it on her lap. We pull our chairs closer. Intricate diagrams, symbols, and explanations. It's even color-coded. My spine tingles, my whole body shakes, and my eyes water. The ladies try to compliment her, but she'll have none of it.

Look at this: my daddy, my Uncle Nate, my Uncle Bix. Over on my mother's side, my Uncle Sweet Pea. And these two here. I can't even remember their names. I never saw any of them anywhere but in prison. Other families had cookouts on weekends. We went to prison.

Look down here. These are my brothers. Ben, Jimmy, Reg. I drove up to Huntsville and visited them Sunday.

This is me and my sister. My sister—see this "X"? That means she's dead. Dorothy's body jerks uncontrollably in the chair for a few moments. Then she regains control.

My sister coughed up her lungs right on the kitchen floor. Right in front of her two children. A child shouldn't have to see his momma die like that. I had to go in there and clean that up. By myself, in this chair—my brothers were too busy doing dope and robbing people. That was my own sister's lungs I cleaned up. She had TB.

My sister was what you call the family symptom-bearer. I looked that up in the book. And Dr. Holleman says I am the glue—the one who holds the family together.

The group tries to tell Dorothy how much they admire her, but she will have none of it. She doesn't want our pity.

Are you angry? somebody asks.

Huh? Dorothy looks confused.

You don't talk about yourself—at least until today. I figured you were angry at the rest of us for not having to suffer the way you have.

Why would I be angry? Dorothy takes a moment to look each lady in the eye. *Getting shot saved my life. At that time I was killing myself on crack. Being in a hospital six months, in total retraction—I couldn't move. I couldn't do dope, neither. But that's not what I want you to help me with.*

Everyone in the group leans forward.

What I want to know is: why my momma never gave her love to me. She NEVER gave her love to me. Ever! My daddy and my brothers never did shit for her, and she couldn't love them enough. My sister was a dope fiend, and Momma nursed her like a baby. I was the only one, other than my momma, who could take care of herself. When I was a child, I'd go up to her and say, "Momma, I love you." I'd put my arms around her and try to hug her. She'd just stand there, hands at her side, like I wasn't even there. Then she'd say: "Oh, you go away girl." Or: "Girl, what is wrong with you?" Why … Dorothy struggles to complete the sentence. *Why did she treat me that way?*

Dorothy—tough, strong Dorothy—balls like a baby. She goes on and on, snorting and shaking in her chair. It's a scary sight—is she having a seizure? Everybody gets quiet. Except Nika.

Oh my God!

We all bristle when Nika speaks up. She's a free spirit, and she's about to spoil Dorothy's breakthrough moment.

I know why your momma treated you that way!

Dorothy jerks up straight in her chair. She's as alarmed as we are. What?

Your momma knew you were the one who would become the backbone of the family. Just like she was. She was making you strong.

Dorothy sits there, poker-faced, saying nothing.

Nika continues: *She wanted to hug you and hold you, but she loved you so much she knew she had to make you strong. And she was a good momma, 'cause you ARE the backbone of your family.*

Dorothy rubs her eyes with the back of her spastic hand. There are no tears; it looks like she's scratching an itch. *Are you saying she treated me this way BECAUSE she loved me?*

Nika smiles.

Dorothy speaks, but to herself, not the group: *I am the backbone. Just like my mother.*

After a while, Dorothy emerges from her trance and reconnects with the group. With tears dripping onto her blouse, she looks around at the group, jerking her body from left to right so she can see each woman without moving her chair. She stares deep into their eyes, and now they stare back, no longer nervous about the jerks and spasms. *Ladies, I thought I would take this to my grave.* She relaxes. And so do we.

Then Dorothy goes back inside herself for a moment: *Of course! Of course my momma loved me.*

Suddenly she seems soft and warm, satisfied and approachable. She has become one of us. Her facial expression hasn't changed, but it feels as though she's smiling with her whole body. We all just sit there and relish the moment.

But I'm still stuck on something they said a couple of minutes earlier. *Backbone. The backbone of the family.* What a metaphor! I'm dying to underscore the profundity of Nike's insight.

Several times I start to say it, but something tells me to keep quiet. This is their group. It's not the metaphors that they need to deal with, but the reality.

Note: This is a true story from many years ago. All names have been changed to protect the privacy of the clients.

Ashley Mann

Breach

I wish I had seen you on your first voyage, years
ago, sturdy and unremarkable, sailing gleefully to the
horizon. By the time I saw you
the great storm had raged itself apart
and you needed repair.
But everything began to break down,
leaking, listing, steadily failing. Bacteria turned to
ballast in your brain, the rotting bilge of your
kidneys. They crusted your heart
like barnacles. Then one morning
you were adrift, dead of becalming,
and when I ran to you
you were flawless, a tenderly
loved vessel, never more magnificent,
and your family wept, unhelmed, asking
what kind of fate could leave the most perfect part of you
behind.

Air

On the screen black bubbles glided down the staff
of your femur, gripping your tibia. I scrolled

noiselessly through the images
again and again. We smiled

at your jokes and pushed your bed
down to surgery a few hours later—

you would have strolled in
if we'd allowed it.

In the operating room I adjusted
my gloves and listened for the wet gasp

I knew I would hear when we released
the balloon of your muscle,

like a newborn drawing breath
for his first plaintive howl,

but between the lowing mumble of the surgeons
and the droning hum of the bone saw

I couldn't hear anything at all.

Watching The Fire Trucks Gather above Highland Road

The poets stood
at the base of the burning hill
and took notes.
Everyone was safe

so they rooted for the fire.
They understood the need
to burn not for warmth
but light.

LeeAnn Bartolini

Note to a Suffering Patient

I have lived inside dirt,
a close companion of Persephone.
Traveled through hollow channels of deep, boggy soil—
decomposing material burying us beneath.

I have lived on top of blossoms,
a lover of Rudbeckia, Ranunculus.
Studied mystery, magic, miracles—
fluffy sailing like a swan.

From a barren barrack in the Gulag
to the plush playing field of riches,
I have learned one lesson—you will survive
and at times—thrive.

Modernity/Post (a Nod to Robert Hass)

Imagine a bar without a name.
Imagine, waiting, alone.
Silly, flirty conversation with a Physicist—
and then
a lecture on String Theory
you pretend to comprehend.
And when you slept that night

the Black Widow spider and the grieving woman in Katmandu and the plastic bottle
you placed in recycling today and the gunshot in the Congo and a veiled child at
school in Paris and a quilt being stitched in Alabama and a bulb bursting through the
hardened earth of that country where they wear those funny wooden shoes and the
conception of a goat and the drop of a rock in the smoky waters of an Alpine lake all
connected when you wake.

Poetry of Aunts

As she lost her mind
she thought with images, smells, not words

Today it was the color of dry earth absorbing rainfall
and tomorrow
the smell of two matching eggs over-easy simmering in vinegar
—it did not matter

Sometimes she recognized the sensation before you need to scratch
as a cotton candy machine twirling sugar
or
she saw the curious shape of her old thumb curled like an angry rattlesnake

Earthquakes are common in San Francisco she was once told, but today she could
not remember this
as the earth quivered beneath her back
lying in the tall grassy field over the hill in Nicasio

Amanda Skelton

Attack of the Killer Calories

Back in the 80s, when I was a medical student, a professor told our class that of all the "scopes"—stethoscope, microscope, laparoscope, colonoscope, to name a few—the one most useful in making a diagnosis was the one the medical suppliers didn't stock: the retrospectoscope. Magnifying lenses, earpieces that transmit sound, fiber optic tubes that can snake into the darkest depths of the body: none of these compare with the ability to look back with the 20/20 vision of hindsight. This has proved to be the case with my son's illness and, in fact, my life.

Sometime in 2002, Riche, my eleven-year-old son, was jumping on a trampoline at a friend's house. I was sitting on a veranda with the other mother, sipping herbal tea—peppermint? chamomile? I don't remember. It was late afternoon—a warm, sunshiny day like so many other days in Mullumbimby on the north coast of New South Wales. The air was filled with the sound of children's laughter and a floral patchwork of smells from the garden. Suddenly, Riche called for me. His voice was loud. He sounded as if he was in pain. I ran to the trampoline and found him cradling his right wrist. "I think it's broken," he said. One minute, Riche's arm was fine; the next there was a sharp crack in his radius, the thicker bone in the forearm. We got x-ray films to confirm the fracture and plaster to protect his arm while the bone healed. No dithering on my part (is it broken, bruised, sprained, a neurosis?). No desire for me to cast blame (the darned trampoline!). No endless search for the cause (the darned trampoline!). And six weeks later, Bob's your uncle and Riche could get back on the trampoline.

Anorexia wasn't like that. It couldn't be diagnosed with a simple laboratory test. It masqueraded as other things: a get-fit program, a desire to eat "healthy" foods, a love of animals that led to vegetarianism, a concern for the environment, yet another example of quirky behavior in this child of ours with a frighteningly high IQ and a sensitivity that made him weep at things as disparate as road kill and the US invasion of Afghanistan. And like middle age and dental plaque, it crept up on us over time.

The seeds of Riche's illness were probably already sewn on that sunny day when he bounced off the black, springy surface of the trampoline and flew, for brief seconds, into the air, feeling the rush of warm air against his skin, the freedom of overcoming gravity, and the strength and suppleness of his young body, before he came crashing down and felt the searing pain as his forearm connected with the hard metal frame.

Brisbane, January 2003

Discombobulated. That's the word that best describes how I felt. Like one of those weird dreams where you suddenly find yourself naked in the street or peeing in public. But this was no dream. Instead, it was the last place I expected to find myself with my eleven-year-old son—outside Footprints of Angels, an eating disorder clinic in Brisbane, two hundred miles north of our home in Mullumbimby, where I'd left my other two children, nine-year-old Andy and six-year-old Louise with their father.

Riche looked at the high brushwood fence as if it enclosed a gulag. "I'm not going in there," he said. "You can't make me."

I hesitated for a moment. It didn't look like a clinic. Instead the fence, unmarked letterbox, and discrete side entrance gave it more the appearance of a brothel, a place where people came and went unobserved, a place of secrets, a place with stigma attached. I opened the gate.

"In we go." I tried to sound purposeful. I tried to act as if I didn't feel like my skin, stretched thin and tight over my body, was the only thing holding me together. My son flicked his ash blonde hair off his face and shook his head, his expression blank, unreachable, a will-o'-the-wisp. He was dressed in one of his anorexia uniforms—a blue Mambo T-shirt that hung from coat-hanger shoulders, light gray trousers (a child's size 8) that showed the abrupt angles of his hips and the bony knobs of his ankles, and brown leather sandals that he could scuff on and off without undoing the buckles. These were trusted clothes, clean and calorie free.

"It's here or hospital." I wanted my words to sound like a reminder, but there was no mistaking the threat in my voice. Riche was showing signs of cardiac compromise. His pulse rate had dropped. He got dizzy when he stood up. He was at risk of sudden death from cardiac arrest.

Riche knew from the look on my face that he had no choice. He let his long fringe fall forward, like a veil, and shuffled through the gate. I followed him into a small but well-tended garden. The scent of jasmine and gardenias, rich and cloying, hung heavy in the air. A patch of neatly mown grass was on our left. On our far side, an old jacaranda tree shaded a picnic table. To our right stood a classic Queenslander house, built high off the ground on stilts. The downstairs area had been enclosed and when I looked through the window, I could see comfortable seating and a large work table. We made our way down a red brick pathway to a staircase along the front of the house that led up to reception. The creak of the steps under my feet could have been the sound of my fear. This was my son, my firstborn!

The building's exterior might have resembled a house of ill-repute, but the interior was straight out of a suburban beauty salon. Calming shades of pink, powder blue, and pale lemon covered the walls, and the sofas were awash with chintzy cushions. Angel figurines reclined on the desk, perched on the bookshelf, swung from the door knobs, and eyed me insouciantly from the coffee table. A host of angels, all female. Not an Archangel in sight. More discombobulation.

Riche scowled as he took in the estrogen-charged surroundings. A receptionist confirmed our details and asked us to wait. I took a seat at the end of a sofa under the serene gaze of a crystal angel. Riche shuddered and remained standing. Nothing I could say would shake his belief that previous visitors—meat-eaters perhaps—had carelessly littered the sofa with calories. If Riche sat down, these microscopic cluster bombs of energy would infiltrate his skin and colonize his cells, and he would swell like the fly-infested carcass of a cow. Rather than risk this, he paced back and forth, burning calories. A victory march for the disease that sucked the life from him.

Wraithlike girls with perilous clavicles and concave bellies drifted through the room, their footsteps mere whispers against the dark wooden boards. They were all teenagers, older than Riche; they were all girls. Horrified, I stared at them, at their skinny bodies, at their tight, pinched expressions. Controlling, manipulative: medical school stereotypes wormed their way into my consciousness. I started up out of the chair. Riche didn't belong here. But his body told another story. As he circled the perimeter of the room, stopping only to allow one of the girls to pass, he looked as if the smallest of pushes could knock him to the floor. He was one of them; the stereotypes were wrong. I settled back on the sofa and concentrated on the steady in and out of my breath.

The click of heels sounded in the hallway, and a woman appeared. She looked a similar age to me—mid to late forties—but was a glossier version of womanhood with the self-assured air I associated with women whose physical attributes—blonde hair, generous breasts—attract attention. Another mother, I thought, but anyone could see from her bright cotton print dress and her blow-dried hair that her daughter wasn't as sick as Riche. Caring for him left me with neither the time nor the energy for mascara or nail polish, and my crumpled shirt, faded jeans, and the dark roots at the base of my unruly blonde-streaked curls smacked of self-neglect. The woman looked at me and offered a lipsticked smile.

"I'm Jan." She held out her hand. "The Director."

The feeling was of something—the fragile scaffolding of hope—collapsing inside me. Jan wasn't the suit-attired professional I had expected. She looked more like a lady who lunched, and she looked like she made a habit of it. How could she help my son? Yet again I chided myself. The stereotypes were rolling off the production line. Jan deserved a chance. I scrambled to my feet and shook hands.

Jan asked us to go with her to the green room. This was a place big on color coordination. A green fabric angel, too flimsy to work miracles of any kind, hung from the green room door. Inside, the dim lighting and the frenetic floral of the green upholstery gave the room a vaguely threatening feel. Riche loitered near the door. His enormous blue eyes, their light dulled, darted around the room.

"It's safe to sit down, Riche," Jan said. "The chair won't hurt you."

Jan's words instilled a measure of comfort in me. She understood Riche's unvoiced but obvious fears. Riche glared at Jan but perched next to me on the sofa, away from the cushions. Who knew how many calories lurked among those ruffles? Living with an anorexic was, I found, like living in France: a few months of immersion and you became fluent in the language.

A young woman sat in an armchair in the corner of the room. Her face had a fresh, scrubbed look, and her hair, almost as blonde as Jan's, was tied in a high pony-tail. Jan introduced her as Sonia, one of the therapists.

Jan turned to Riche. "Why did Mum bring you to see me?"

Riche shrugged and looked at his feet. I shifted in my seat, desperate to find the angle from which Riche's silence did not look like denial. When I had made the appointment, the receptionist had told me the clinic only took patients who accepted that they were sick. This didn't make sense to me—wasn't denial a characteristic of the illness?—but I didn't get to make the rules. And now it looked like our game was up. But I kept quiet, not wanting to be one of those parents who speaks for their children. My resolve lasted a good three seconds.

"He's lost weight. He won't eat."

Jan nodded and leaned forward. "You're emaciated, Riche." She spoke in a no-nonsense voice, almost cheerfully. We might as well lay the facts on the green (yes!) table. "Perhaps Mum can tell me what's been happening."

Curiously, while I had long since thrown out my medical school teaching of the controlling, manipulative temperament underlying this illness, I continued to hold to the teaching that Kevin and I were the classic parents of an anorexic child. Somehow we had screwed up. This belief was aided by a Methodist upbringing that left me only too willing to assume guilt. So I offered up every argument, death, dietary quirk, and relocation that came to mind. Viewed through the retrospectoscope, it looks like circumstantial evidence. At most, it's only part of the story.

"Does he really have anorexia?" I said when I'd finished. Still, with the evidence sitting right there beside me, hope, an unreliable emotion, bloomed.

"A classic case," Jan said without a second's hesitation. "But you and Kevin aren't to blame. Having an anorexic child doesn't make you a bad parent."

Not a bad parent. Out loud, the words had a hollow ring to them, like the sound my knuckles make when I rap on the gas bottle if the kitchen stove won't light. In addition to my medical training and Methodist upbringing, there was the obvious factor that Riche wasn't raised in a vacuum. Surely there needed to be some reckoning of his childhood. Furthermore, if we didn't cause Riche's anorexia, who or what did? This question would continue to haunt me with damaging consequences for many months, years even. If only someone had told me that blame looks like ugly great shackles around your ankles. It drags you down, hobbles you, makes you a prisoner of your own doing. Not my fault? Not Kevin's? For now I said nothing.

Jan turned to Riche. "I know you have a voice in your head that says you're fat, but it's lying. We call that voice the negative mind. Can you hear it?"

Riche shook his head. I steeled myself for the inevitable rejection.

"We can offer Riche a place in the program."

"But you don't take people in denial."

"In this case, we will. Riche is on the verge of acceptance, and because he's so young and so sick, we need to act. It's a race against the clock."

Jan told me that Riche needed a weekly program of four counseling sessions with Sonia and one session with the nutritionist. I said we'd start with two counseling sessions and did he really need to see a nutritionist? Jan said yes. I said I couldn't see the point for an eleven-year-old boy. Riche didn't prepare the meals; I did. And ignorance about calories and nutrition didn't seem to be the problem. Quite the reverse. He read energy charts and food labels like a professional. Jan said something along the lines of the nutritionist working to improve Riche's relationship to food. I thought bullshit. But I said yes, which just goes to show I didn't understand the basic principles of consumerism. Or that I was scared witless.

Jan went on to tell me that I would be excluded from Riche's sessions and would not be given any feedback. Here I lost the thread of logic. Why the need to exclude me if I were not to blame for Riche's illness? Especially when he would be in my care 23 hours a day. Asking him to eat a cheese and Vegemite sandwich was akin to asking my husband to eat steak with cyanide sauce. I needed help. Instead, I would be left to steer in the dark, sidelined to the roles of cook, chauffeur, and cheerleader. Not if I could help it. I would educate myself. Borders and I were about to embark on a close relationship. Nonetheless, I was grateful to have found a place where Riche would be treated with compassion while living under my care.

Compassionate treatment came at a price. Each session would cost one hundred and ten dollars. The Day Program that Riche would be unable to attend because of his fear of footloose calories would have cost an additional fifty dollars per day. Protein powder for supplementary shakes, if needed, cost forty dollars per week. Our private health fund would cover the nutritionist's appointment but not the counseling sessions. The cost to attend full time amounted to seven hundred and fifty dollars per week, in a country with a free public healthcare system, albeit one with big black holes such as an outpatient support facility to treat anorexia. Not exactly a bargain, but we could afford it. I would have sold my soul or my body, whichever fetched the higher price, to get Riche back, the happy healthy Riche.

We moved on to logistics. Would I move to Brisbane? No I wouldn't; I had two other children. Didn't I think the trip would tire Riche? And how would he control his negative mind without Sonia's daily coaching? I would see how we went. *If a twenty something year old with a twelve month counseling course under her belt can do this, why couldn't I, a doctor with six years of training,* is what I thought. *And who would help Riche on weekends?*

"What about school work?" I said.

"No school." Jan's voice was firm. "Riche needs all his energy to fight this illness." The right advice but the wrong reason as I would discover.

"How long will this take?"

"It could take five years, longer even."

I closed my eyes and let myself sink into the blackness behind my lids. My body felt heavy and lumpish. Five years! This disease would rob Riche of his childhood. He would never again "watch with glittering eyes the whole world around" as Roald Dahl's narrator urges in *The Minpins*, a book Riche's godmother had given him. How would he discover "the greatest secrets" or find "the magic"?

I looked at Jan. "Anorexia is going to change our lives, isn't it?"

"Forever." Jan returned my gaze without smiling. "This illness can break up marriages."

Marilyn Morrissey

Cycling

It was mid-September, 2004. Summer was swiftly slipping into Fall. Just the three of us were home now—me, Jim and Julia. Sean, our oldest son, was living with roommates in an apartment in Somerville and working part-time as a clerk at Harvard. Glen was a sophomore in college up in Maine. Julia, our little girl, was a 9th grader and an "only child" for the first time in her life.

She was fretting about the fact that she couldn't ride a bicycle. Well, technically she could (I had taught her a couple of years earlier) but we hadn't practiced since then and now she had no confidence in her ability. It was suddenly a big issue because she was considering various teen travel programs for the following summer, including a month-long bike trip. No matter how many times I reminded her of our successful attempts to get her up on two wheels and the fact that we still had plenty of time to practice before the trip, she would not be reassured. "Why haven't we gone biking?" she demanded. "You went biking all the time with my brothers!"

Why indeed. The accusation hung there in the air. It was true. We used to go biking all the time with the boys. They had spent their babyhoods being driven around town in a bike seat on the back of either my bike or their father's. When Julia came along, the same was true for her for awhile and, by that time, the boys were riding their own bicycles. We had even bought a special cart to attach to Jim's bicycle to haul her around through her toddler years. We called it her "magic chariot" and, for a few years, until she got too big for it, we continued biking as a family. But, then something happened. Our biking lives ended.

I can trace it back to the summer of 1996 when Julia was six years old. Jim had been laid off from his medical executive position and tensions had mounted. Raising three school-aged children had become more complicated and stressful. I was working part-time as a clinical nursing instructor, making very little money, after I had been laid off myself from my Nurse Practitioner job. Relations between us had become strained and we began drifting apart, even as we continued to live together as a couple and raise our children.

Over time, Jim got new jobs and dived whole-heartedly into the new work challenges. I turned to community work, serving on boards and volunteering in the schools. He became a soccer referee and devoted his weekends to his new passion. It seemed we had less and less time for family activities such as biking. In this way and in other ways, we had failed our daughter. Her inability to ride a bicycle at age fourteen indicted us.

Jim came home from his soccer game late that afternoon in his silly referee uniform. I confronted him as soon as he walked through the door. "She doesn't know how to ride a bike! She's fourteen years old and she doesn't know how to ride a bike!" He was feeling satisfied after a good game and had been trying to feel more optimistic since we had seen the cardiac surgeon in August. All summer long, he had prepared himself for mitral valve repair, explaining his increasing fatigue and shortness of breath on his prolapsed valve. He worried also about the one-time sugar spill in his urine, picked up by his PCP during a routine exam. But I swatted away his worry as a fluke, perhaps a lab error, asserting that the sugar could not be replicated and, anyway, his follow-up serum A1C was normal. Then the surgeon had reassured us that Jim's prolapse was not yet bad enough to justify open heart surgery and had told him that he could continue reffing for now. But he wanted Jim to bring his blood pressure down to take some of the pressure off his leaky valve and had ordered some new medications. I had to admit that I was feeling a lot of relief that he wouldn't be having the surgery, as much for myself as for him. Truthfully, I dreaded having to take care of him for the three month rehab. Although I was a nurse and a mother and the eldest sister in a big family, a natural born caretaker, I didn't want to take care of him. Throughout our marriage, whenever he became ill, which wasn't often, I became angry and anxious. Threatened somehow.

"Well," he said, feeling magnanimous, "I think we need to correct that situation right away!" "Now?" I blurted out. "It's almost five o'clock!" "No time like the present time," he replied cheerfully, still pumped up from his game. "We still have a couple of hours of daylight left." "But, our bikes have been in the shed for years," I emphasized the word bitterly, "they're probably all rusty and flat." "A little oil and air will fix that," he said, heading up the stairs to change out of his uniform. A few minutes later, I heard the back door open and his steps descending the stairs towards the shed.

I was flabbergasted and suspicious. He wasn't usually one for spontaneity. But I decided to go along with his mood, to suppress the bile bubbling up in my heart. Maybe he was trying hard to convince himself that nothing was really wrong, that his fatigue was due to simple aging or overwork and not due to something more nefarious. Maybe he was trying to make a new start and spend more time with his shrinking family. Maybe, perhaps, he was just trying to please me.

Through the window, I watched him consumed by his task in the backyard. He had the three bikes on their backs and was busy with his tools adjusting gears and patching tires. He had always had that ability to lose himself in a task, a single-mindedness that I both respected and resented. He was wearing the old khaki shorts and camp shirt that I loved so much. He looked like a fit, handsome, aging, bearded, Boy Scout. I saw the light beginning to fade in the sky and worried that the magic of the moment would be lost. Finally, he came in and said that the bikes were ready to take off.

We set off slowly on the bike path behind our house towards the Arnold Arboretum and the setting sun. We lined up like a family of ducks—Jim, protectively at the front, Julia in the middle, and me, taking up the rear. Julia was wobbling between us but with each stroke the lessons learned years ago began to return to her legs. Within a few minutes, we were safely at the arboretum gates and away from the streets and traffic. The air was warm, the trees were beautiful, the sky was red and the old pleasures of riding together filled me up with hope. We pedaled leisurely back and forth around the flat sections of the park. The light was getting low so we decided to stay off the hills this time. There would be more time for that another day, we promised our daughter. We had the whole rest of the Fall and all of the coming Spring to get her ready for a possible summer bike trip next year.

Delighting me further, Jim suggested that we all bike the short distance to Centre St. for dinner instead of riding straight home. Over the years, our main street had gone from rough-scrabble, working-class, grated storefronts to a mix of gentrified chic restaurants and stores. The sushi fare at JP Seafood was one of our neighborhood favorites. Carefully, in the twilight, we escorted our daughter along the city streets and locked our three bikes together to a pole outside the restaurant. We went in triumphantly and ordered the same dishes we always ordered—scallion pancakes for her, agedashi for me, and spider maki for him. I sipped on a glass of plum wine and enjoyed the warmth washing over me. I was happy. Our new, little family constellation had enjoyed an outing together and there was the promise of more such times to come.

Night had fallen while we dined so I suggested that we take the small hill behind the restaurant home, a short-cut off the main streets and through a quiet neighborhood of stately homes and lightly-traveled, one-way streets. We urged Julia up the hill, "Keep pedaling—don't stop!" and celebrated her struggling success. She fell behind us as Jim and I rode slowly side-by-side chatting amiably as we crested the hill along a strip of parked cars. I was enjoying the quiet evening and the effort of my legs and thinking about the love we might make later on that night. The sound of a car engine accelerating behind us startled our attention away from ourselves and back to our daughter. In synchrony, we quickly turned our heads to the left and to the rear.

Julia was safe, the car had spotted her and slowed down but in our sudden, jerky movements, Jim's front wheel had caught mine and we both went tumbling down to the pavement. He was always such a klutz! Tall and gangly, our marriage was full of his legendary, almost comical falls—other biking accidents crashing into curbs or parked cars, broken ribs from a fall on a frozen pond, walking into and bouncing off a glass door in a fancy restaurant and so on. But this time the fall was gentle and I got up with only a small scratch on my calf and without uttering a cruel word. Jim was still sitting on the ground under his fallen bike and squished up against a parked car. I picked up his bike and offered him a friendly hand. "My ankle is broken," he stated matter-of-factly, nodding towards his right leg, waving off my hand. "It is not!" I protested. "How could it be?" "I don't know, Marilyn," he said, "but I can tell it's broken." And that's when I saw it for the first time—he looked old and frail slumped there on the street.

Why was he doing this to me? I wanted to wail to the heavens! First his heart, now this! When had this shift happened? Is this when the seven year age difference between us would come into play? It had never seemed to matter before—not when we first became lovers when I was twenty-five and he was thirty-two. Not when he was forty and I was thirty-three or when I was forty and he was forty-seven. But, now at fifty-one and fifty-eight, suddenly he seemed so much older than me. I felt sick to my stomach. When had he forgotten our unspoken pact? He was supposed to take care of me and I would take care of everyone else. That's the way it had worked for years. He was the one who wasn't supposed to leave me, not even if I asked him to, not even if I tried to push him out the door. "Oh, come on now, Jim, get up!" I pleaded, staring down at him.

Behind me, Julia pulled up with her bike, and a man, a stranger, ran out of his Victorian house to help. They both pulled Jim up as I stepped aside, frozen and ashamed of my inaction and lack of sympathy. While Jim leaned back on a car balancing on one leg, the man offered us all a ride home or to the hospital. "No thanks," said Jim, shaking his hand gratefully, and mounting his upright bike with his good leg on the pedal and the other one dangling by the side. "We can get ourselves home. It's all downhill from here."

I pedaled behind him as he glided down the other side of the hill towards home, his lame leg bouncing limply by the right side of his bicycle. Behind us, Julia tried nervously to keep up. When we pulled up to the front of the house, Jim dismounted and, standing on one leg, asked me stoically, "Could you put my bike away in the shed? I want to go in the house and get off of my feet." "What do you mean, get off your feet?" I hissed. "We're going to the hospital!" "No", he said, laying his bike down on the sidewalk and hop-scotching to our front steps, "not tonight." "It's

Saturday night and the ER will be bombed. I'd rather just rest and ice it here and go in the morning." "But, what if it's dislocated?" challenging his medical judgment. "It's a simple fracture," he responded, "it can wait a night." "How do you know?" I grumbled out on the sidewalk. "Do you have x-ray vision now?" "Marilyn," he replied, I thought rather condescendingly, "relax. It's only a fracture; it's no big deal. It can wait. I'm tired. I just want to lie down right now."

No big deal! I felt furious and flummoxed. How could he be so calm? I knew what this would mean. It would mean that I would have to do everything for the next several months—all the chores around the house and all the errands. Everything! And how would he get to work? Easy for him to say it was no big deal!

Jim turned and hopped up the front stairs, pulling on the rickety wrought-iron banister rail. We have to get that fixed, I thought, before someone kills himself. It was another thing on our long list of things that needed fixing around the one hundred year-old house that we had lived in for twenty-one years. And now, Jim would be even less available than usual to tend to that list.

Resigned, I put the bikes away with Julia's help. "Don't worry," I said to her, "Daddy will be fine. And, you and I can still go biking." By the time I had gone into the house through the back door, Jim had hopped or crawled up the stairs to our bedroom. I found him there lying on our bed with his broken leg propped up on a pile of pillows. Somehow he had managed to take his sneaker off and I saw the injured ankle swelling inside his tight, white crew sock. "You'll cut your circulation off," I said as I peeled off his sock. The skin was shiny and purple beneath my fingers. It didn't look good. "Can you make me up a couple of ice bags?" he asked solicitously. "And can you bring me my *Times* and my laptop and a couple of ibuprofen?" And that's how it began—my nursing him, fetching things, adjusting my schedule to his needs, like I had done for each one of our three children, only more willingly.

The next morning, still fuming, I was relieved when our oldest son agreed to take his father to the ER for the x-ray. A few hours later, they returned home— Jim now in a knee length, non-weight bearing cast and teetering on a pair of tall crutches. "No dislocation," he announced cheerfully, "just a simple fracture of the fibula, should heal in six to eight weeks." "Great," I groaned, "glad to hear it." This was not the way I wanted to spend the Fall, our favorite season, the autumn of our twenty-fifth wedding anniversary. I had secretly looked into a return to that old farmhouse inn in the White Mountains where we had honeymooned so long ago. I had hoped that maybe a weekend of hiking along the same foliage-strewn trails would recapture those times and feelings and strengthen our bond. We hadn't been away alone since our twentieth anniversary when we had biked together all over Martha's Vineyard. But we wouldn't be hiking or biking now, not this year.

We would just have to find another path back to that special place, some other way, some other time, if we could.

It began with the car rides. Jim had always been the first one up in the house, bolting out of bed without an alarm at 6:00 AM and downing a quick breakfast of All-Bran, the cereal the kids called "sticks." He left the house precisely at the same time each morning, jogging down the street to the subway station to be the first one at work. He timed it perfectly so he could be at his desk by 7:30 AM before his staff arrived. He believed in punctuality and, as the head of his medical department, he felt he had to set a good example. "I can't criticize them," he said, "if I come in late." And so, since I worked part-time and didn't have to be in until ten, I began driving him back and forth to work after he broke his leg. Spending those ten to fifteen minutes together each morning started a new pattern between us. After pulling on a long, white, tube sock over his cast to keep his toes warm, we would set off driving the city streets past all the familiar sites between our house and the hospital where he worked. Sometimes, we chatted a little but much of the time we rode quietly observing the people and daily activities along the way.

There was the tidy, little man in his black leather jacket sprinting down the street towards his subway stop, his tiny white earplugs obscuring his hearing and perception of the traffic around him. "Dangerous," my husband would pronounce. "A Mack truck could run him over and he'd never know what hit him." "Or a mugger," I would offer, recalling the time that Jim had been mugged walking down our street reading the *New York Times*. How outraged I had been at him then for not paying attention to his surroundings!

There was the same gaggle of school kids and their distracted, tired moms in various stages of housedress, waiting at the corner for the yellow bus to take their children away for the day. As the days and weeks passed, the only thing that changed was the added layer of clothes and coats piled on as the weather cooled. There was our friend and neighbor, "Tiny," the tallest man we knew, riding his gigantic red bike towards the high school where he tried to teach employable shop skills to insolent teenagers.

It went on like this through the season as Jim's leg healed. I began to look forward to our little commutes. He often rested his left hand on my right leg as I drove. He admired my finesse with short-cuts that avoided traffic and delivered him to work in minutes. He appreciated my help and the extra sleep he was getting in the morning. Getting out of the car, he would peck me on the cheek before hopping away on his crutches with his old, leather backpack slung over his right shoulder, the one I had given him for his 40th birthday. In the evening, I would pick him up at the street corner across from his office and we would reverse the route home.

We explained away his increasing fatigue with the obvious efforts involved with ambulating around home and work in a heavy cast and crutches. His blood pressure continued to be higher than desired despite the change in medications, which frustrated and worried him. The cardiologist had set a goal of 130/70 but it remained stubbornly intractable in the range of 140/90. Jim went to bed right after supper each night, exhausted and needing the rest.

One night in October, while propped up by pillows behind our backs and under his wounded leg, side by side in bed, reading separate medical journals, I came across an article about renal arterial stenosis, a narrowing of the renal artery that can cause chronic hypertension. "I wonder if you have this," I mumbled half-heartedly, not expecting him to consider it seriously. "Easily diagnosed with a CT-scan," he responded. "Well," I carefully ventured, "maybe you should get one, you know just to rule it out." He was a conservative physician, not one for ordering unnecessary medical procedures, interventions, or treatments, including the latest pharmaceuticals, hawked by Big Pharma. So I was surprised when he took the bait. "Good idea," he replied. "I'll call my cardiologist tomorrow and ask him to set one up." I was pleased that he thought my idea worthy but understood that he was worried now about how he was feeling and he wanted some answers.

Two weeks later, in early November, a few days after the CT-scan had been conducted, Jim called me at work. I was alarmed when I heard the weakness in his voice and even more alarmed by his request. "Can you pick me up?" he asked. "I don't feel well and I want to go home." Never in all of our years had I known him to leave work early! He had accumulated hundreds of unused sick days over the years. Hurriedly, I drove the fifteen minutes from my office to his with a feeling of dread. I spotted him standing on the familiar street corner, leaning on his crutches, looking exhausted. I pulled over and he opened the car door and slid in, collapsing in the passenger seat as he tossed his crutches over the back seat of the van. I waited, holding my breath. "My cardiologist called this morning with my CT-scan results," he reported softly, almost whispering. "He said my kidneys look great," sighing, "but he says there's something on my pancreas." Instantly and instinctively we both knew we were doomed as the missing puzzle piece fell from the sky into place. Jim patted my knee. "Somehow, we'll get through this," he promised.

But, I could not be reassured nor hear his voice nor feel his hand. I could only hear the sound of the other shoe dropping, the one I had been waiting for my whole life. I was not thinking of Jim, at that moment, nor of myself. I had already left my body and traveled across town to our beautiful, innocent daughter sitting naively at her schoolhouse desk, ignorant of the disaster about to befall her. Hovering above her, I imagined her future laid out in front of her as mine had been. Like her mother, she would lose her father at fourteen, fixed in that time frame forever. Like me, she would grow up scarred and full of grief, unconsciously equating Love with Loss. She would be unwilling to give herself wholly to another, to expose her vulnerability to someone who would only hurt her and desert her in the end. She would be marked, always on the look-out for danger lurking around every corner and within every loving relationship. She would be unable to love her husband enough to keep him healthy. Like her mother, he would leave her and she would be alone.

Jan Haag

Grow

Your death, when it finally arrived,
was not wall after wall of crashing waves,

but a single body blow—
air leaving me so fast

I had to sit down.
I counted my heartbeats,

tried to reel in breath
with your bamboo fly rod,

the one on which you'd snagged
your first fingerling trout.

I still have the picture pinned
to our kitchen bulletin board—

your teeth like stars behind
broad lips, shades blotting

your eyes, the spotty fish
gleaming in your palm.

I saw you let it go, saying,
"Grow." As I cast for air,

I felt your steadying hand winding
the line, the leader, the caddis fly,

the same hand that stroked my thigh
before sleep. I heard the rumble

of your voice, *Great gams, Toots.*
And, as the laugh

lurched up my throat—
breathe.

Night Watch

From my bed, I hear the cat bring it in—
soft plump of a furry body dropped
to the floor, tiny nails scrabbling to flee,
a pounce. I sigh, tap on the light,
feel my feet hit hardwood.

She sits, head bowed,
looking at her downed prey—
small and gray, long black tail curled
into a C. I can see it breathing hard,
imagine the staccato of its heart,
this possum-playing mouse.

As I reach for a towel to scoop it up,
hoping to return it to the night,
the mouse springs, scurries
to temporary safety behind the bookshelf.

The cat looks up at me.
"Your fault," I hear her think.
"You're right," I say.
We both study the wall of books for an answer.
She settles down for the night watch.

I know how this ends.

I go back to bed, knowing one heart
will stop beating in my house tonight,
knowing I cannot save this one little life,
as I could not save yours.

Aphasia

Sidelined on a gurney,
alone in an ER hallway,
she reclines, eyes closed,
lashes moist, lips dry,
her bulk swathed in pink.

All her words, newly formed
as a fetus, lie trapped in her brain;
her lips try to form foreign letters,
push syllables through broken synapses
to scrubs-clad people she identifies
as "pretty hair" or "that guy."

She believes all the lost words
lie stored in her liver,
which will never be able to speak.

Oh, to send rescuers down
into the cavern of her liver
on long ropes to retrieve
words from the dark.
She would air them out,
proudly display them
as the lost artifacts they are.

Sarah Paris

This Body Sings with Despair

Out of the depths
of its blackest wounds
from the broken bones
marking its wilderness
a voice cries out:
"Life is a blessing!"

As I walk in the shadows
at dawn, the song sparrows
call to the sky: alive!

At sunset, my homeless neighbors
beat their drums in the park,
shouting their love.

When darkness falls,
I rage against God; my angel
brother whispers: Fear not.

Awake in the dead of night
the sound of the fog horns
pulls me back into the sea

of sleep, where a small
wave of courage carries
me across, once more

to welcome the cat
stretching and sweetly sinking
its little daggers into my flesh.

Questions I Must Never Ask of My Mother

What did you say when you broke the news to *your* mother?

Who washed off the blood stains, you or my uncle?

How did you comfort my five-year-old brother?

Have you ever talked about it since?

Do you understand why I miss him, even though I never knew him?

Do you think of him with love, or hate, or not at all?

Do you remember his voice?

Do you remember the way he made love to you?

Did he say good-bye to you before he shot himself?

Have you forgiven him?

Have you forgiven yourself?

Was he really my father?

Will you tell me any of these things before you die?

Going Down

Switzerland is known for its neatness,
clean toilets and the punctual departure of trains.

My ancestors were farmers there, kept trim borders,
collected each apple that fell from the tree.

But I love the color Verdigris, which arises
when copper is weathered, exposed to the elements.

And I'm at ease exposing a man's body,
kissing his scratchy chin, his sweat, his balls,
while the sight of my hidden parts makes me recoil.

Underneath the silky sheets, we all find shelter.
Giddy like children, we play games in the dark,
our reptile tongues darting in and out
of furry rabbit holes.

Sharon Dobie

from the John Fox Sessions

For Michael

If I sit with your life
laughing while you sleep towards death
remembering cartoons and fears and comedy
that worked together
weaving who you are,
I will not deny you led me
and I will dance inside my heart.

Even to This

Even to this,
there must be
should be
will be homage.
Even to this,
intention or running
or wily pretending
will not suffer the space
where even to this
is known.
No longer a silent appendage
or adjective denied,
I will welcome the nowhere else
that brings me out.

Daylily

Let my mind wander.
Let my hands play.
Let my feet meander
in those lilies
whose prolific blooms become stingy
as the sun settles the day.

Good Enough

His disheveled appearance and shuffling gait sharply contrasted with the purposeful walk of the bike-helmeted professional in pressed jeans from only six years earlier. It was a visual reminder of a process I could not seem to impact. I wanted him to get better. It did not matter who made him better. It could be his work, the efforts of his other doctors, the medicines, or some twist of fate as unexpected as whatever put him in this shadow state. Doctors can be hard on themselves. I can be hard on myself. It is maybe easiest to feel good about our work and who we are when our patient gets better, gets over the illness, is fixed, cured. In this case, I didn't need to be the effective one. I simply wanted him to be well. His not improving was linked to my dread when he was on my schedule.

When I first met him, he was a project manager in a growing technical field and said he would soon be promoted. He rode his bike everywhere, despite an old knee injury, saying "of course I ride; more people should ride for our environment and my knee actually is better when I keep it moving." He was married with three children, sharing that he did half of the childcare, was a room parent at school, coached a soccer team, and loved helping his kids with their homework. I never saw him in those places and could only rely on how he talked about his life and activities. In those early encounters, his voice was confident and his mood seemed calm when he described a life that appeared engaged and thriving.

He came to me in search of more effective relief of pain from the old knee injury. Every few months we laboriously reviewed the materials from prior evaluations. He carried a bulging file of x-rays, MRIS, physical therapy reports, and orthopedic, pain, and neurology physician clinic visits. These records from the other doctors all agreed on a diagnosis of osteoarthritis. The main clues to a deeper anxiety and compulsion were the frequency of his visits and his reluctance to accept that his prior evaluations and treatments had been both informative and exhaustive. Each time he came to see me, he would ask, "Might it be something else? Are we missing something that could be made better?" Although he said he lived with daily pain, he also said it did not affect or limit his work or physical activity. Citing time and cost reasons, he declined the physical therapy, massage, and acupuncture I offered. He said he only wanted to know what was wrong. He seemed to need constant reassurance that it was not something worse. I asked about his mood at most visits, and he insisted he was fine.

"What do you think it is?" I would ask.

"I don't know. I just want the pain to go away. I want to know what is causing the pain."

We would again review all the tests that had been done and whether more testing was needed. "You seem to worry. Are you kind of anxious?" I asked.

"Pain gets you down, ya know. I don't like to not be able to move around without pain. And I worry that I have a bad disease. Sometimes I am a little depressed." I suggested counseling and antidepressants; he declined them.

About two years into our relationship, he developed new symptoms of abdominal and chest pain. A treadmill, some blood tests, and an ultrasound were reassuringly normal. Pain continued to be the main theme of our discussions. Most of the time it was his old knee pain. Sometimes it was the chest or abdominal pain or a new pain, always pain, always physical pain. Often he rated it at eight out of ten, with ten being severe pain.

With further discussion, he admitted to feeling sad and dejected on more of his days. He denied most other symptoms we associate with depression, including any thoughts of harming himself or someone else. Though he adamantly held to the belief that the pain was the problem, he agreed to work with a former counselor of his and to take an antidepressant medication. In a subsequent visit, he said he was feeling much better and that the counseling was helping him to feel calmer.

Then over the next few months, he appeared to literally unravel. He came to one appointment frowning and would not sit down. His speech was rapid and his blood pressure was elevated. As he paced around the tiny exam room, hands never quiet, he admitted to stopping his antidepressant and said that he and his wife had separated. His voice rose as he said that he had asked for a transfer to a different section in his office and that the response was to terminate him. "I am going to file for unemployment and fight the termination," he said. "OK so I have had my mind on other things and have not gotten all of my work done. I will look for other work." As his pacing increased, I felt my blood pressure rising. His rapid, loud, emphatic monologue continued for several minutes.

When I was able to interrupt, I asked him about his medications and why he had stopped them. I asked him if he had thoughts of hurting himself or others. "I have no interest in hurting myself. It is my pain; that is the problem. I won't discuss this any more. It is always the same pain. I will be fine if you will just take my pain away!" he kept insisting. At this visit, his pain was in his hip and groin. He said he could not afford physical therapy and massage, so I suggested some exercises for him and we discussed a regimen of daily medication. I stressed how concerned I was about his emotional state, recommending that he restart his antidepressant medication and have a consultation with a psychiatrist. He agreed to see his counselor the next day, to consult with a psychiatrist, and to reconsider medication.

I saw him several times soon after that. Despite his psychiatric care and medications, he became a shadow person within what seemed like days and was likely months. I could hardly see in him the person I had known and I would not have recognized him on the street. His clothes became wrinkled and his hair uncut. His posture stooped. His voice became so quiet that he seemed to be disappearing into himself. All he would discuss was his pain. "I will be fine if you will make this pain go away. I am in terrible pain all the time." We reviewed all his prior tests and repeated some. I reinforced his work with psychiatry. He was back on an antidepressant and seeing his counselor, but he said he had no relief from his pain.

I shared my thoughts. "I can't tell you what part of your pain is from the arthritis and what part is because you are depressed. What I do know is that when you are depressed, like you are now, you will feel your pain as worse. It is real pain. The treatments are the exercises, staying active, taking the medications, and then really working hard with your counselor and psychiatrist to resolve your depression." We tried medications for the pain and he agreed to resume physical activity. At this point I felt anxious for him and I was still hopeful that his care would bring him out of his depression and help his pain.

At an appointment a few weeks later, he became agitated, started pacing, and told me he had made a grave mistake and could not forgive himself. "I am ashamed of what I did and I deserve to feel guilty." He disclosed that his pain was worse when he was feeling guilty. "I betrayed my family and I cannot live with myself," he said and he would not tell me more. Our Mental Health Professionals offered him voluntary admission that day, which he declined. They did not think he was in imminent danger of self-harm. The next day he went to the emergency room, talked of ending his life, and was hospitalized.

After being discharged from the hospital, he moved with reticence, became uncommunicative, and wore his depression with a frightening countenance. Some of it was the medication and some seemed to be the expression of his current emotional reality. He seemed three inches shorter. Each step he took was small and tentative, like a person with Parkinson's disease. His hands now moved with a tremor and could not be still. His face looked immobile, empty, and expressionless, like a face in a wax museum. It was as if he put on a costume for a theatrical role: "Now I am a depression and there is nothing else to me."

He was hospitalized a number of times over the next several years. Usually a suicide note found by his son or a method or plan found by his wife precipitated these hospitalizations; occasionally he just knew he needed to be in the hospital. His children kept going to school, but told their mom they worried all the time. His wife went to work and they all worked with a counselor. Yet who knows what the outside world really understood about this family? Only occasionally did it seem as if the medications and work with the psychiatric team were effective. In those periods, his pain was also better and he got back on his bike and was active. Even then, after a brief interlude, the symptoms of his all-consuming delusional guilt would return and he would again say his pain was worse, that he felt paralyzed, and he was thinking of ending his life. He would be readmitted for medication adjustment and counseling and then discharged after anywhere from days to weeks. He met with his mental health team every week or two and came to see me once or twice a month.

That is my attempt to tell his story as I saw it, the parts he let me see and hear, my rendition of his story. And there is more of course. There is all I cannot know about him and his story. And then there is our relationship, because I was his doctor, which of course influences how I tell his story and the story of our doctor-patient relationship. Early on, I felt like the second opinion doctor, reviewing the extensive work of others, helping him to understand what the reports said, reassuring him, and encouraging him to stay active and take occasional over the counter medications. Our conversations felt amiable and collaborative to me, even with his many worried questions and appointments that lasted longer than the allocated fifteen minutes. Yet, I worried that I would not be able to help this man; his pain was not improving and he did not ascribe to any emotional or stress related triggers. I sent him to other specialists and hoped they would find something I could not see. I felt anxious seeing him on my schedule because while I thought he left feeling cared for, I never felt he left feeling helped. Those knot-in-my-stomach pressure-in-my-head feelings that generally signal that there is more to the story in this case alerted me to this man's severe depression.

During the last couple of years, I dreaded seeing him in clinic. Although I knew he was not in control of his illness, I was frustrated and upset with him. Why couldn't he, why didn't he take control and just get better? Of course I realized that my anger was really because I was unsuccessful in changing the course of his illness. We did discuss reasons to live, including his love of his wife and children. Once we talked about a prior suicide gesture and the impact it had on his children, who had become anxious and hyper-vigilant. "How can you even contemplate suicide?" I asked. In my mind, having children all but removed that choice from a menu of options.

I struggled to control my feelings and not to convey judgment. He swore, "I am not going to end my life. I just cannot live with this pain. If you want me to live, take away my pain." Could I take away his pain? Medications, joint injections, other therapies when he could afford them had no reliable effect. His pain, believed by him to be specific to his muscles and joints, was to me the barometer of where he was with his psychiatric illness. Reflecting outside of our visits, I feared for his life; he had, in theory, the best psychiatric and medical care available. Yet none of us had taken away his pain.

I received the page in the middle of a busy clinic. It was the lead psychiatrist from his team telling me that he had committed suicide. He had not kept an appointment, which was unlike him. They requested a safety check and found him deceased. I was not really surprised by the news; in some ways it is numbing to fear a potential event for years. I wanted something different for him, for his family. He was in his forties when he took his life and I was his doctor for most of the seven years before that.

I wonder: did I do enough for him? Could I have done more? I believe the answer is yes and yes, both answers contributing to the disquiet within me. His magnified and delusional guilt and self-loathing provided me with a lens for reflection about my own sense of guilt and inadequacy. Along with my sadness about his family's loss, I also had to recognize that my anger and frustrations were as much with my limitations as they were with him for threatening and then carrying out his suicide.

Doctoring gives me ample practice in exploring those ambiguous and shifting lines about responsibility and at least approaching a compassionate place with myself. How is it that any of us humans come to understand that maybe, just maybe, we are good enough? How many lessons that require self-assessment and then forgiveness must we have along the way towards that understanding and acceptance? All of our care did not keep him alive. Even when my efforts do not yield what I would want, even if my efforts fail, even if. Some days these are what we have: the effort, the even if, and the good enough.

Terese Svoboda

Compassion in Fiction: Can't Get Enough of It

> For ourselves, are not each of us the center of the universe?
>
> William Carlos Williams, *The Doctor Stories*[1]

First a compassion joke:

A man was sitting on a blanket at the beach. He had no arms and no legs. Three women were walking past and felt sorry for the poor man. The first woman said, "Have you ever had a hug?" The man said "No," so she gave him a hug and walked on. The second woman said, "Have you ever had a kiss?" The man said, "No," so she gave him a kiss and walked on. The third woman came to him and said, "Have you ever been screwed?" The fellow said, "No." She said, "You will be when the tide comes in."

My perception of your profession is that you are forced to run through flames. You either burn up or wear those thick, ropey scars from those fires for the rest of your life. Touch is arbitrary, tentative, painful. I want to talk about compassion for you in literature, and by you—and how that relates to being a writer.

Compassion, according to my lousy Word dictionary, is a sympathy for the suffering of others, often including a desire to help. Medically, compassion is the result of being unable to help any longer, it happens when you have to throw up your hands, it appears at the intersection of desperation and imagination.

It would seem that all caregivers are drawn to the medical field out of compassion—you want to help however you can—but you know as well as I, the reasons are often more complex. Perhaps some of you have experienced primary trauma at some point in your past, which led you to being attracted to the field, perhaps you are the type of person who is especially attuned to others which makes you excel at your job. Either way, we laymen expect caregivers to be skillful and compassionate—not *House*.

---

1   William Carlos Williams, *The Doctor Stories*. (New York: New Directions, 1984).

The stereotype of a writer is *House*: analytic, godlike, and arrogant about his gifts. However, writers who portray the world outside themselves must have empathy and the ability to see modulation in motives and behavior beyond what they themselves can personally experience. Good writing requires compassion in order to create complex characters, select appropriate points-of-view, project acceptable turns of plot arising from the conflicting motives of characters. In addition, writers, like physicians, often teach and that skill also requires abiding compassion. Teachers of writing are not just red-penned critics of grammar and punctuation but also act as caretakers of important matters of the psyche and trauma that require compassion.

Let's start our literary case studies with the modernist master-and-doctor, Chekhov. He revolutionized the short story partially as a result of his medical training, which relied upon his compassionate eye. When he outlined his choice of form and substance for his own work in a letter to his brother Alexander, these were his tenets:

1 Absence of lengthy verbiage of a political-social-economic nature;
2 Total objectivity;
3 Truthful descriptions of persons and objects;
4 Extreme brevity;
5 Audacity and originality; flee the stereotype;
6 Compassion.[2]

In stories like "The Grasshopper" (1892), "The Darling" (1898), and "In the Ravine" (1900)—to name only three—Chekhov reveals much compassion in his subtle humor and irony. The concreteness, impartiality, empathy, compassion, and diagnostic acumen in his stories also arise from and/or are consistent with his medical sensibility and training. Likewise his focus on the individual rather than the grand scheme.

Let's have a look at a brief quote from "In The Ravine."

---

2   Anton Chekov. *The Cambridge Companion to Chekhov*, ed. Vera Gottlieb and Paul Allain. (Cambridge England: Cambridge University Press, 2000), 61.

There was something new, something gay and light-hearted in her
alms-giving, just as there was in the lamps before the icons and in
the red flowers. When on the eve of a fast or during the local church
festival, which lasted three days, they palmed off on the peasants
tainted salt meat, smelling so strong it was hard to stand near the tub
of it, and took scythes, caps, and their wives' kerchiefs in pledge from
the drunken men; when the factory hands, stupefied with bad vodka,
lay rolling in the mud, and sin seemed to hover thick like a fog in the
air, then it was a relief to think that up there in the house there was a
gentle, neatly dressed woman who had nothing to do with salt meat
or vodka; her charity had in those oppressive, murky days the effect
of a safety valve in a machine.[3]

Chekhov describes the woman's charity by opposition—showing the callousness
of the villagers toward the drunken peasants who have come to celebrate a festival.
The accurate details that describe the workers—rolling in the mud—and their pledges,
particularly their wives' kerchiefs, give Chekhov authority, that is, given the minutae
of the details, the reader trusts him to know the broader picture, even the interior
lives of these characters. Like the woman in the story, Chekhov doesn't judge the
peasants or look down on their activities—they just occur and will occur, and will
always require compassion.

Eudora Welty wrote about compassion directly in many stories but most notably
in "A Worn Path." It's about an elderly black who woman walks to town for medicine for her grandchild. As she totters through the forest, Welty's description and the
woman's commentary allow the reader to come to know her courage, cunning and
dignity. Here's a quote:

At the foot of this hill was a place where a log was laid across
the creek.
"Now comes the trial," said Phoenix.

---

3   Anton Chekov, "In the Ravine," *The Portable Chekhov*, ed. Avrahm Yarmolinsky. (New York:
Penguin, 1977), 464.

Putting her right foot out, she mounted the log and shut her eyes. Lifting her skirt, leveling her cane fiercely before her, like a festival figure in some parade, she began to march across. Then she opened her eyes and she was safe on the other side.

"I wasn't as old as I thought," she said.

But she sat down to rest. She spread her skirts on the bank around her and folded her hands over her knees. Up above her was a tree in a pearly cloud of mistletoe. She did not dare to close her eyes, and when a little boy brought her a plate with a slice of marble-cake on it she spoke to him. "That would be acceptable," she said. But when she went to take it there was just her own hand in the air.[4]

Later in the story, Phoenix is greeted by the clinic workers, who recognize that she's come for medicine for her grandson who had swallowed lye several years earlier. They deny her dignity. She's seen as poor, "a charity case," stupid, and greedy.

"No missy, he not dead, he just the same. Every little while his throat begin to close up again, and he not able to swallow. He not get his breath. He not able to help himself. So the time come around, and I go on another trip for the soothing medicine."

"All right. The doctor said as long as you came to get it, you could have it," said the nurse. "But it's an obstinate case."

"My little grandson, he sit up there in the house all wrapped up, waiting by himself," Phoenix went on. "We is the only two left in the world. He suffer and it don't seem to put him back at all. He got a sweet look. He going to last. He wear a little patch quilt and peep out holding his mouth open like a little bird. I remembers so plain now. I not going to forget him again, no, the whole enduring time. I could tell him from all the others in creation."

"All right." The nurse was trying to hush her now. She brought her a bottle of medicine. "Charity," she said, making a check mark in a book.[5]

---

4   Eudora Welty, *The Collected Stories of Eudora Welty.* (San Diego, NY, London: Hartcourt, 1980), 143.

5   Welty, 148.

Welty could have written a fuller description of the lives of the clinic workers—the nurse with two kids who fight all the time or the doctor with a drug problem, in order to express compassion toward their situation as well but the economy of effect provides the reader with the writer's assessment.

Compassion is useful in writing about other cultures. Harriet Doerr does this well while describing the superstitions of the Mexican people in her book of connected stories, *Stones for Ibarra*:

> "I have found this thorn," said Sara, "and I have also seen the crack in the blown-glass lamp. I believe the thorn was placed there to prevent me from noticing that the lamp was damaged."
>
> Lourdes said nothing.
>
> "I am sure it was an accident," Sara went on. "Perhaps it happened when you were reaching for cobwebs with the long broom. All of us sometimes break things. What I cannot understand is your belief that this thorn could keep me from finding out."
>
> Lourdes turned down the flame and covered the pot. She faced the American woman.
>
> "It is true that the thorn failed to prevent your disappointment," said Lourdes. "But señora, consider this. The engineer and the geologist who visited here a month ago succeeded in finding the means to keep the mine from shutting down. Then don Ricardo himself let it be known that he had received good news from the bank. And as you will remember, the senor recovered quickly from his recent illness. All of these things happened while the thorn was on the lamp."[6]

The Mexican woman is allowed to explain the efficacy of her practices so the reader can decide for himself their relevance to his own set of beliefs.

Later on in the book, Doerr describes the situation of a Mexican doctor who commits suicide partially as a result of the strength of superstition overwhelming his skill and compassion: "To the doctor it must have been like emptying the sea with a thimble. The pregnant Acosta child wearing that belt of corn. Victor and his raw alcohol diet."[7]

---

6   Harriet Doerr. *Stones for Ibarra*. (New York: Penguin, 1984), 1 1 1.

7   Doerr, 1 3 1.

The doctor can't reconcile his work among people who refuse his services. He had only compassion to offer, which was soon exhausted in the frustration of having the means to cure them being rejected.

Joy Williams writes compassionately about a cleric in a hospital where his wife is a patient. The story is "Taking Care," the title story of her 1985 collection. Here is the opening paragraph:

> Jones, the preacher, has been in love all his life. He is baffled by this because as far as he can see, it has never helped anyone, even when they have acknowledged it, which is not often. Jones's love is much too apparent and arouses neglect. He is like an animal in a traveling show who, through some aberration, wears a vital organ outside the skin, awkward and unfortunate, something that shouldn't be seen, certainly something that shouldn't be watched working. Now he sits on a bed beside his wife in the self-care unit of a hospital fifteen miles from their home. She has been committed here for tests. She is so weak, so tired. There is something wrong with her blood. Her arms are covered with bruises where they have gone into the veins. Her hip, too, is blue and swollen where they have drawn out samples of bone marrow. All of this is frightening. The doctors are severe and wise, answering Jones' questions in a way that makes him feel hopelessly deaf. They have told him that there really is no such thing as a disease of the blood, for the blood is not a living tissue but a passive vehicle for the transportation of food, oxygen and waste. They have told him that abnormalities in the blood corpuscles, which his wife seems to have, must be regarded as symptoms of disease elsewhere in the body. They have shown him, upon request, slides and charts of normal and pathological blood cells which look to Jones like canapés. They speak (for he insists) of leukocytosis, myelocytes and megaloblasts. None of this takes into account the love he has for his wife! Jones sits beside her in this dim pleasant room, wearing a grey suit and his clerical collar, for when he leaves her he must visit other parishioners who are patients here. This part of the hospital is like a motel. One may wear one's regular clothes. The rooms have ice-buckets, rugs and colorful bedspreads. How he wishes that they were traveling and staying over-night, this night, in a motel. A nurse comes in with a tiny paper cup full of pills. There are three pills, or rather, capsules, and they are not

for his wife but for her blood. The cup is the smallest of its type that Jones has ever seen. All perspective, all sense of time and scale seem abandoned in this hospital. For example, when Jones turns to kiss his wife's hair, he nicks the air instead. [8]

Compassion means you, the writer, arrive at the party knowing nobody, happy to be out of the house, grateful to be introduced, and open to all the guests and their eccentricities. Compassion in a story makes the writer look good. Without compassion, the reader may sense the writer is looking down on him, either in omnipotence (the reader knows nothing) or by looking down at the story's characters (they are fools). The reader also likes to feel that he has some say in how he interprets a story. Although the writer must maneuver his scenes, his diction, and his world of characters to achieve an effect that might release certain emotions in the reader, he doesn't like to feel manipulated. No forcing. If the reader senses the writer wants him to get out a hankie before he's ready, then by god, the reader will resist. Of course the writer will always know more than the reader about the characters and the situation—he controls the narrative—but he must release this information in a way that allows the reader some play, some reading between the lines, some space for the reader to understand himself in the writing. Readers have their own opinions about how people relate and emote, just as—if I might attempt a comparison—the patient has opinions about his illness and will try to diagnose himself. Like the writer with the reader, the physician needs to use compassion to secure the cooperation of the patient in order to get information about his condition. Patients are not experimental laboratories, not marks to push products on, nor are they intentionally being difficult communicating their problem. Treatment, like the experience of reading, is a give-and-take relationship, a partnership. The more informed the patient, the better the conversation between him and his physician, and likewise the reader and writer. The writer has to be willing to explore not only the evil side of the villain but the good side as well, or at least the side that has become crippled over time and accounts for his aberrant behavior. God and zombies, for that reason, are boring. Too one-sided. They have no complexity of motivation, no possibility for compassion. The reader need not care what happens to them and must only read for plot. If this lack of compassion is unintended—no zombies or God—and the characters act only to benefit the plot, the whole enterprise becomes unconvincing. Perhaps this is similar to what happens

---

8   Joy Williams, *Taking Care*. (New York: Vintage, 1985), 10.

when a physician has no time for compassionate listening and makes an incorrect diagnosis, fitting the patient to the wrong plot.

Being a pitch hitter, doing both fiction and poetry, I also have a few words about compassion and poetry. In order to form a "compassion aesthetic" for poetry, I had to wade through the inspirational. This did not happen as frequently in fiction. Why is that? Reader's Digest swallows inspirational stories? The narrative form demands blood and guts? Redemptive memoirs fence in the inspirational? Perhaps poetry is expected to be about sad situations, the poor me ballad. But when poetry thinks about something other than itself, it can invoke the compassionate.

Ironically, Whitman's *Song of Myself* is the ultimate celebration of compassion, embracing all and everyone in the 19th century, including Buddhism, as part of himself.

> Walt Whitman, a kosmos, of Manhattan the son,
> Turbulent, fleshy, sensual, eating, drinking and breeding,
> > No sentimentalist, no stander above men and women or
> > > apart from them,
> No more modest than immodest.
>
> Unscrew the locks from the doors!
> Unscrew the doors themselves from their jambs!
>
> Whoever degrades another degrades me,
> And whatever is done or said returns at last to me.[9]

---

9   Walt Whitman, *Song of Myself*. (Stillwater, KS: Digireads, 2006), 30–31.

A lot has happened in the world of poetry since Whitman, but let me suggest that there now exist two camps: the compassionate and the less compassionate poets. We will start with the more difficult, the less compassionate, who are the language poets, those who vow not to comment about the nature of one character's reaction to experience. However, even Charles Bernstein, the *jefe* of the language poets, sometimes approaches compassion. Here is the end of his six page poem "Dysraphism" (a term for a kind of birth defect):

> Dominion demands distraction—the circus
> ponies of the slaughter home. Braced
> by harmony, bludgeoned by decoration
> the dream surgeon hobbles three steps over, two
> steps beside. "In those days you didn't have to
> shout to come off as expressive." One by one
> the clay feet are sanded, the sorrows remanded.
> A fleet of ferries, forever merry.
> Show folks know that what the fighting man wants
> is to win the war and come home.

The great language-poetry explainer, Albert Gelpi, states that the poem's "verbal play avoids or disguises interpretive comment or constructive patterning because such impositions would suggest a center of perspective, attitude, response—in short, all that is dismissed as the lyric ego of the Romantic-Modernist poet."[10]

Who are these Romantic-Modernist poets? Gelpi names Roethke, Lowell, Berryman, Olson, Duncan, Levertov, Rich, Berry and Snyder. They are poets who believe that even in the face of the violence of contemporary history, the word can effect personal and social change, that poetry can, almost against the odds, make things happen—psychologically, morally, politically and religiously.

---

10   Albert Gelpi, "The Genealogy of Postmodernism: Contemporary American Poetry," *Southern Review*. Summer (1990): 517-541.

Raphael Campo, a wonderful poet and director of Harvard's Program of the Medical Humanities, wrote on the limits of compassion in writing:

> It is impossible to know entirely the experience of another person's suffering. To suggest otherwise, even in a discussion of the great empathetic medium of poetry, is another kind of hubris. So if I write a poem about my deaf patient, I don't   become deaf myself, nor do I even approximate the experience of deafness. It's the gesture toward the possibility of mutual understanding that is so necessary, the reaching out, especially coming from the perspective of biomedicine, which so actively imagines the opposite—that there is no value whatsoever in contemplating deafness, just get the sign language interpreter or adjust the hearing aids and move on. I think instead poetry asks how we can all be implicated in an individual's experience, and thus how can we best be of service, how we can best be present, mindfully, emotionally, at this difficult moment but stop short of saying glibly, "I feel your pain."[11]

All teaching requires compassion, but writing in particular exposes the writer-student more personally and directly to the teacher than other disciplines. Sometimes when I will find a student who is choking on his story or poem, suggestions from fellow students only serve to further tamp it down inside him or else twist it into some more acceptable form, rather than allowing it freedom to fulfill its intentions. If, despite dreadful grammar, atrocious spelling, cartoon characters, stereotyped scenarios, a teacher senses that the student is struggling to say something important to him, he can guide the writing to honor the student's intentions so the student may yet learn to write what he must.

The following is a story about my lack of compassion, and the grace one student had to grant me another chance. A couple of years ago I had a roomful of teenage refugees whom I told to write about their "most forgotten memory." It was foolish of me to attempt this with such a traumatized group. My assigned task was to have them write the story of their lives for a bulletin board. I wanted them to write something deeper, something more meaningful. My assignment released all kinds of violent stories, one that resulted in a very big Mexican boy covered with tattoos asking to

11   Raphael Campo, "Of Poetry and Medicine: Raphael Campo in Conversation," interviewed by Cortney Davis. *Poets.org*.

leave the room with the implicit suggestion that he was going to get a weapon. I refused. And he refused to tell me what he had been writing. Only after class did he did he tell me about his brother who died in his arms of gunshot wounds in a gang fight. He had wanted to leave the room in the middle of class to cry in the bathroom.

Compassion among students is also required for useful writing feedback. A reader must look at what the writer has tried to accomplish and praise that first—when the writer is still listening. It's human nature to try to block out criticism. It takes quite a while before the comments or the scrawled red marks really make sense. That's true even for me, with years and years of red marks. It is also important to honor the separation between the writer and the writing, however autobiographical the work may seem. Criticism should be supportive and aimed at the work, not the writer. The writer is only the vehicle for the work, just as the patient is only the host for AIDS or cancer.

Having compassion for yourself and for your subjects as caregivers, you can use the terrible burns you've suffered from your profession in writing. You can picks at the scabs, showing how awful they are, or else write how you understand my suffering by way of yours. Either way, scientific research suggests that writing about emotional distress is good for both body and mind, not in the least because you can step out of your own shoes as a writer. Unless you're an actor or an undercover agent, there aren't many times in your life you can do that. Your voice is separate from your characters' voices, even the most interior first person. In contrast to your professional position as a caregiver, you are not the one responsible for what happens, except in the authorial sense. You may slaughter your sentences and your characters as you wish. There are no malpractice suits in writing.

I'll end with a poem of my own, from my new book *Weapons Grade*:

Three Plucked Ladies

Three plucked ladies chemo-
glutted, cocktail-wavy,
radiate into my kitchen.

Oh, my. Food is beside itself,
dust balls. You've seen
curtains hang?

Even the little threads
fighting the chair
retract when they sit.
But words waft,
heads hum,
bulbs on.

An offering of me,
as generous as that, there is
no other. I want to pray

but it's too late, they've harked
in semaphores, in series,
in sighs a whole meal of

Good Gracious. I hug them well,
their thin selves. I tuck each into
her trauma. I turn my head.[12]

---

12   Terese Svoboda, *Weapons Grade*. (University of Arkansas Press, 2009), 82.

Fran Brahmi

Bumper Sticker

Love your local poet, I said.
I already do, he said.

Remembered

As the ashes scatter
across the great blue
from Malibu to Monterey
I recall:
the Mediterranean
of my childhood.
Like fine pearly dust
floating and sinking
undisturbed;
leaving only
traces of
DNA.

On Losing a Son

Dark black olive eyes
bright and attentive
Snowy-white wooly hair
Cool ebony nose

Perky as a pup she once was
And even now, while dragging her hind legs,
always ready for a treat.

I knew it was time
and yet
I wanted her to hang on just
a little longer
She was Craig's after all
How could I let her go too?

As we sat in the vet's office
waiting
she fell asleep.
She too must have known
it was time.

Therese Jung Doan

Procrastination

ignoring alarms
    pretending that things
    are under control while
    the house is on fire!

an elephant
    thumping on my chest
    with every breath.
    It hurts like hell!

staying up all night
    thinking but not writing
    let things sit there like
    stale tobacco smoke …

praying and waiting for
    divine inspiration
    which only shows for the faithful
    who choose completion over
perfection.

Time

That time he did not let go of my hands
I'm sorry, I'm sorry
Forgive me, forgive me
He said over and over again

I told him not to bother ...
When my father was murdered
and mother was dying,
and all those times, the yelling and screaming

That time he held on
I'm so sorry, I love you so much
Oh yeah, I have no idea
Then I saw the hurt and the tears

That time I took his hands to my heart
I forgive you, I always love you
We held each other for a long time ...
The last time.

Madeleine Biondolillo

The Virgin Point

My high-school Advanced Placement Biology teacher reverted to her somewhat unfortunate last name after divorcing a man she had married with great fanfare only two years earlier. Miss Butts was lecturing from the front of our musty-smelling science room on the biochemistry of cellular energy production. It was early one Friday morning, a month before our AP exam. During her marriage, Miss Butts had become Mrs. Sirna, but clearly not wishing to be defined by her marital status, she now insisted we call her Ms. Butts. It was rumored that she had applied to medical school.

"The Krebs Cycle is the first stage in the process of cellular respiration, which turns the glucose in the food we eat, and the oxygen in the air we breathe, into energy," began Ms. Butts. "This chemical energy is called adenosine tri-phosphate, or ATP for short." She paced the floor as she spoke.

"ATP molecules provide the energy for all the important processes in our bodies. Things like flexing the muscles necessary for us to breathe and contracting our cardiac muscle so that our hearts beat. The waste products of this cycle of chemical reactions are carbon dioxide and water, which we exhale and pee out." Someone in the classroom giggled.

Studying my biology text the night before, I learned that Hans Krebs had garnered the credit for working out The Citric Acid, or Tri-Carboxylic Acid, cycle that was a series of enzyme-catalyzed reactions. I thought, how cool that the acronym "TCA" fit both names. But after a long week of anxious studying wedged between softball practices and my after-school grocery store job, I was not expecting anything really transcendent in the biology realm. The seniors had told us that the Krebs Cycle was a bear, and definitely going to be on the test, and I was lamenting missing my train that morning and with it the cup of coffee that represented energy production for me.

The science lecture room was also our laboratory, so our biochemistry apparatus was visible as my mind wandered temporarily away from the lecture, and I peered off over the Bunsen burners and beakers assembled on the benches in front of the windows. My eyelids drooped heavily for a few moments as I gazed toward the sunshine streaming in through the glass. Briefly, anxiously, I was pulled back to my recurrent dream of the past few years in which my parents angrily stood up from their seats in the small Quaker meeting room in which we sat in a circle on Sundays. Each strode off in the opposite direction in continued silence, though not the introspective, awaiting-the-Spirit silence I knew was expected of us. My father, raised Lower East Side Ukrainian Jewish, and my mother, raised Jew-distrusting Polish Catholic, had both converted to Quakerism while students at Columbia. My early sense of confusion about religion had become magnified during their bitter divorce until it had expanded into generalized confusion and anxiety. I respected the Quakers for their noble quest to find "that of God in every man," but I knew that I wasn't one of them. The squeak of the chalk was wrenching.

Ms. Butts was getting very excited about her subject matter now. We could tell because she was pacing quickly and flailing her arms as she went. I sensed something important coming.

"Cellular respiration is a complex process involving dozens of steps to break glucose's six carbon structure first into pyruvate, then citrate, then succinate...." As she lectured, she stopped mid-molecule, and drew the beautiful, complex-yet-simple, circular diagram on the board from memory.

"... and finally back into citrate. This releases the phosphate necessary to produce the energy molecule, ATP!" She turned to us, beaming.

I felt a rush of caffeine-less warmth flow through my body and sensed, without understanding what was happening, that her energy, Kreb's energy, the TCA cycle's energy and very likely some even more powerful and important energy were in that room and flowing through me. I was electrified with excitement, contemplating the perfection of this life-giving energy production. At the same time I felt a strong sense of peace because of its perfection. At that moment, our world seemed guided by a loving, orderly, ingenious, and altogether miraculous presence.

Many years later I was a participant in a writing group comprised of women who had survived domestic violence. For a long time I had struggled with self-pity and rage at the brutality I suffered at the hands of my ex-husband. I told my biology moment story to one woman in the group who happened to be an Episcopal priest. She confided to me that she'd had her own revelatory moment at age five, under a covered table with some Ritz crackers and grape juice, while her parents celebrated Happy Hour. She had felt the presence of God; it was her true first communion. I sensed what her moment had been like and tried to describe the comparable feeling I'd had in the biology classroom at my moment. "I just knew, then, that there was God. I felt overwhelmingly that if the Krebs Cycle was the way it was, there had to be God. The feeling was euphoric. I felt joyful and serene, and I was aware that something important was happening to me."

She said, "Oh yes, the moment when everything's moving, yet everything's still. *Le Point Vierge.*"

In his book, *Conjectures of a Guilty Bystander*, the monk Thomas Merton described his revelatory moment, his sensing of *le Point Vierge*—the Virgin Point. "In Louisville, at the corner of Fourth and Walnut, in the center of the shopping district, I was suddenly overwhelmed with the realization that I loved all these people, that they were mine and I theirs, that we could not be alien to one another even though we were total strangers. It was like waking from a dream of separateness, of spurious self-isolation...."

"... *le Point Vierge* [I cannot translate it, says Merton]. At the center of our being is a point of nothingness which is untouched by sin and by illusion, a point of pure truth ... which belongs entirely to God ... and if we could see it, we would see these billions of points of light coming together in the face and blaze of a sun that would make all the darkness and cruelty of life vanish completely...."

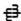

We biology students had heard that Ms. Butts got divorced because her ex-husband had abused her. One day while working after school at the grocery store, I'd seen her wearing dark sunglasses over a black eye while she bought supper for one. Another day, thirty years later, while grocery shopping, I'd wear my own dark sunglasses over a black eye that my ex-husband gave me.

I was so proud when my AP Biology teacher was accepted into medical school. It felt like a pathway for me too, as I got a high grade on that dreaded AP Bio test and eventually also went into medicine. But I remember Ms. Butts most because she taught me to trust what I love. Her passion for her beloved chemical cycle opened my eyes and my heart to the ultimate possibility. In her classroom I came to believe that we each have a brilliant point of light inside us, capable of making all the darkness and cruelty of life vanish completely.

Elizabeth M. Ackerson

Close As I Can Stand

No shower now.
Not much sleep last night
My body shifts its weight
I cannot shed my skin.

Clear the bathroom mirror
mistakes multiply.
"You look good" rings hollow
when again I cannot find

my teacup and my book
the red shoe
in my left hand
the watch on my right wrist

as close as I can stand
to not being present
in my body
in this land.

3 Haiku

Each morning
more smudged away the white moon
through my bedroom window.

Frustrated bumblebee
buzzes into me
touch and go.

Such stillness
pain your body knows
to welcome.

Crossing to Safety

I stood wedged in dirt
between the iron dumpster
and the rhododendron.

The doe stood
splay-legged
on the concrete drive.

Abby Caplin

Morning at Esalen

The spill of morning light over the
Shoulders of the mountain
Onto feathering trees that
Hug the rocky coastline
Pockets of settled fog
Nestle into steep crevasses
Exuberant splashes of white
At the edge of deep blue water

The earth turns
The sun rises
Witness to prowling pink flowers,
The winging of swallows and gnats,
My body rubbery after the
Wet heat of the stone baths.

It Sometimes Happens

It sometimes happens,
we lay bare our necks, expose
the gentle pulsations
of the heart
already marked.

Like snake charmers
hiding danger in a basket
that could hold cookies,
they bide their time.

Too late we rouse
to the flash of fangs,
the sting,
venom,
seizing innocence
our confidence swallowed whole,
souls
quivering.

John Fox

POETRY, COMMUNITY AND THE FLOURISHING HEART
Poetic Medicine as a Catalyst for Resilience and Connection within a Hospital Setting

By making us stop for a moment, poetry gives us an opportunity to think about ourselves as human beings on this planet and what we mean to each other.

Rita Dove, US Poet Laureate 1993

People don't listen to understand. They listen to reply.
The collective monologue is everyone talking and no one listening.

Stephen Covey, *The Seven Habits of Highly Effective People*

We often associate the statement "Know thyself" with Socrates
(via Plato), forgetting that "Know thyself" was the major inscription
on the temple of Apollo at Delphi, and that Apollo was the
original god of both medicine and poetry—in Apollo the two
disciplines seamlessly meld.

Jack Coulehan, MD, State University of New York,
Stonybrook, Director Emeritus Center for Humanities
and Bioethics

Earlier this year I was in Newark, New Jersey, at the University of Medicine and Dentistry of New Jersey, presenting Grand Rounds at the invitation of Dr. Diane Kaufman, head of child psychiatry.

In addition to speaking at Grand Rounds I met with a group of patients in the hospital. Participating was a range of generations, people from their 20s to 70s.

Many of these participants were quite ill. Yet, they showed up to meet this poet and poetry therapist.

Our group also included family members, patients and nurses. The room we met in at the hospital is called the PALM room—that stands for Planned Activities Less Medication!

I began by reading a poem based on the Psalms of David from the Holy Bible. This psalm poem was written by Roberta deKay, a woman living with and fighting a very aggressive cancer.

Psalm 13

Oh Lord, I am sinking in despair
    fearing you have forgotten me.

How long will my mind be confused
    and my heart in grief?

Turn towards me, mothering Healer, bring
    light to move from despair before my
    heart closes.

Gently comes your healing hand
    across my mind bringing what was needed
    before I knew myself.

Trust in your mercy opens my heart
    and I realize again your grace.
I am richly renewed.

    Your mercy is deeper than my despair.

In the spirit of the psalmist, Roberta was crying out to God for solace, with faith.

I felt a psalm-like poem would connect with my listeners, who were almost entirely African American and Hispanic, and that this theme of asking for help when one is close to despair would feel real to the situation of these patients, many of whom were quite ill.

My instincts were correct.

I asked people to speak back a line in Roberta's poem that touched them. While it was slow, there were responses as people spoke back lines:

> How long will my mind be confused
> and my heart in grief?
>
> Turn towards me, mothering Healer,
> bring light

The nurses attending this session were also drawn in, with a sense that this poem reminded them of their own "mothering healing" instinct and spirit. We didn't rush. We took our time.

I believe there is something in poetry that is often akin to prayer, like a psalm, just as there are aspects of medicine related to and that must attend to our spiritual selves.

Dr. Rafael Campo, a fine physician poet from Beth Israel Deaconess Hospital at Harvard, recognizes that spiritual and shamanic component of poetry:

> Putting the mouth to words, and by incantation returning regular rhythms to the working lungs, there were the principles by which ancient healers in Native American cultures practiced their art.[1]

Campo says there is something healing about consciously giving a word our breath. This is something indigenous people have known about healing for millennia.

People mirrored back lines or words that spoke to them. We listened to one another, not in a style of chit-chat or chart taking questions or through technically oriented language, but with a sense of deepening care and attention.

---

1   Rafael Campo, *The Poetry of Healing: A Doctor's Education in Empathy, Identity and Desire.* (New York: W.W. Norton & Co., 1997), 167.

Trust in your mercy opens my heart

Your mercy is deeper than my despair.

Silences wove into our listening. Not the silences of boredom, the tedium of being in or visiting a hospital. It was the silence of precious attention. I had won some of their trust.

Together we made a more healing environment. We could explore through a poem the first seeds of connection and invite through our own thought and feeling green sprouts that could infuse us with a felt sense of resilience.

Then I read a poem about listening deeply, about being deeply listened to. Here is that poem which is something that came to me—I hesitate to say that I wrote this poem—rather it arrived early in my training as a poetry therapist, about 1985.

I was working as an intern at El Camino Hospital in Mountain View, CA:

When Someone Deeply Listens to You

When someone deeply listens to you
it is like holding out a dented cup
you've had since childhood
and watching it fill up with
cold, fresh water.
When it balances on top of the brim,
you are understood.
When it overflows and touches your skin,
you are loved.

When someone deeply listens to you,
the room where you stay
starts a new life
and the place where you wrote
your first poem
begins to glow in your mind's eye.
It is as if gold has been discovered!

> When someone deeply listens to you,
> your bare feet are on the earth
> and a beloved land that seemed distant
> is now at home within you.[2]

The questions I asked were these—what is it like for you as a patient, as a person, to be listened to? What did this poem evoke in you? If you could speak a word or two that reflect what you feel about being listened to, what would your word or those words be?

An older man, seated to my left in the circle, with a neatly trimmed grey beard, a black man, who had up to this point looked abstracted, sad, and distant, spoke up quietly.

I say this gentleman *spoke up quietly* and that sounds like an oxymoron, but indeed his quiet and simple words lifted something up powerfully before all of us. His word carried a deep intention and sense of meaning even though he wasn't proclaiming it loudly—he said one word to the circle of people: "enlightenment."

And then he said "… and that *enlightenment* could be conveyed by a person, place or thing and in a variety of ways."

It sounded as if the gentleman's vocal chords and his lung capacity were badly compromised by illness but there was still an unmistakable clarity and directness in his voice that caused us all to lean toward and become more aware of his presence.

His words and voice were like wildflowers coming through the crack in the hospital concrete. It was one of those "whoa!" moments where everyone stops.

This was clearly the start of his poem and a surprise to me and perhaps to others to discover how much attention he had been giving to what was occurring. This poem, our caring circle, had stirred something true and beautiful in him.

And then a visitor of a young man whose utterly bald head indicated he was clearly in the throes of intense chemotherapy treatment, a young Hispanic woman probably in her mid twenties, perhaps his sister or girlfriend, who had been sitting very politely and quietly, suddenly said in a strong voice, "not being listened could cause me to feel invisible, as if I don't exist," but the listening poem evoked for her a sense of "belonging."

This was an absolutely bell-ringing statement and she said it in a confident and composed way.

---

2   John Fox, *Poetic Medicine: The Healing Art of Poem-making.* (New York: Jeremy P. Tarcher/ Putnam, 1997), 177

Another young man, a patient, Eric, tucked into a corner of our room and our circle, said that the words the poem evoked for him were "a sense of caring, a sense of ease."

Eric too had been quiet and looked shy. Even with that shyness, I asked him, partly because his voice was so resonant with a deep mellow timbre (a quality I felt might go unrecognized in this hospital) if he would read the listening poem to all of us.

He blushed but he took a deep breath and read. It was clear people enjoyed his version of saying that poem and I believe he took that appreciation in. Further connection!

It's important to say here how much the nurses joined in and shared from their hearts. They leaned forward with their elbows on their knees. They leaned close to hear their patients. They were at ease themselves, to use Eric's word, to share from their own hearts.

This is the blessing of nurses and nursing, that is, attending to the matter and person at hand, even to themselves.

And so this poetry circle in the PALM room—the room of poems rather than Prozac if I may say so—soon concluded. At that point, with poetic license, I felt a different name for the PALM Room: Precious Attention, Less Medication.

I wondered, as I walked down the hospital hallway to my next group, whether my visit had felt to these patients like someone landing from another planet!

And yet about two hours later I received, via one of the nurses in that circle, a poem Eric wrote immediately after my visit. Here is Eric's poem:

Tell Me Why?

Tell me why people don't talk
Tell me why people don't feel
Tell me why we close off the
gift that God has given us to feel
talk, love and hear. For this is
one force that makes the world
go round. This brings peace to
the heart. If we can just
tell one person why you feel
that way you do!

Eric Fishburne

Eric says it so well: why poetry therapy can encourage connection and resilience.

His poem recognizes how a whole world, which is, after all, rooted in a whole person, how a person's whole world can be changed by "one person" who hears you, hears why you feel that way you do.

Author's note: This one day at the University of Medicine and Dentistry caught the attention of the Director of Patient Services. She mentioned her experience to the Board of Trustees at the hospital and they in turn invited Diana Kaufman, the child psychiatrist who had invited me to present to the Board of the hospital. They decided to begin the process of supporting the expressive arts.

Muriel Karr

Stigma

---

sex // he died in the act of it
sex // I've called it an accident
sex // I've said he was alone
sex // people assume suicide

stigma // I've skirted it

coroner // it was death by hanging
coroner // accidental death by hanging

autoerotic // an entire sexual history

his private	[	my brother	my brother	]	his private
world	[	a former girlfriend confirms it		]	world
	[	(I hadn't known)		]	

his body // nude but for leather accoutrements
his cottage // with chains affixed to the doorway

coroner // autoerotic asphyxiation
me // autoerotic asphyxiation, my brother's cause of death
            (there, I've said it)

warning // what teenagers call the choking game
warning // there's no safe way to do it! nothing foolproof, nothing!
warning // my brother took meticulous care

online // a support group for family members
online // we hide behind the screen

death rate // accurate statistics still hard to come by
death rate // minimum 100 per year in the US, starting at age 16
death rate // 1000 per year, at least, according to the FBI

new thought // my therapist suggests my brother might have been
new thought // extremely happy just before dying
                    (she says this as I'm crying)

Have You Ever Been Diagnosed

as bipolar asked the sleep doctor
who wasn't getting anywhere with me
and I said no

but when I asked my psychiatrist
he said yes
he'd call it soft bipolar

which at that particular time
was a term
my therapist hadn't heard of

but I fretted
and got sad
so she said it was just a label

I was the same person
I'd been the week before
(on the bipolar spectrum, as we both learned)

is that from A to Z
and I'm a C or an F or an M?
I still don't want this label

and when my neurologist said
he didn't see much to worry about
on my brain scan, I had to go back

to ask him, well, what *did* you see?

The Price of Eggs

I have no children because I have no children
I made a choice   Surgery involved

Would you ask why I have no poodle
Would you ask about my thyroid scar

I get dizzy   I forget my phone number
I pee when I'm not supposed to

My migraines alone drive me wild
Do you need to know any of this

I think I'd be a horrid mother
My own mother was perfect

Joanna Steinberg Varone

My King and I

When I first met my King, it was desire at first sight. He was big and strong, and he quickly proved to be a worthy companion with his comforting embrace and non-judgmental manner. The time I spent with my King was minimal at first—just enough to sustain me for another day. My husband liked my King, too, but their relationship was simple, unlike mine and my King's, which began to blossom as my King and I became better acquainted. Ours was becoming a symbiotic relationship, one I began to be increasingly reliant upon.

Coincident with my MS diagnosis, which I received after a year of experiencing increasingly debilitating fatigue, pain, and spasticity, along with enduring an extensive battery of tests, my relationship with my King began to take a strange—and unpredictable—turn. Each day, as I would walk through the door, whether after work or running an errand or seeing one of my doctors, the drive home became difficult to remember, even though it was I who had been behind the wheel. The climb up the stairs to the foyer would take my breath away, but as I'd drop my purse to the ground, I knew that soon I'd be in the arms of my King. I'd peel off my clothes, and as they'd lie strewn across the hallway, I would finally arrive, naked, my King waiting. As I'd stumble towards my King, I would collapse in his warm embrace. And as I would lie there, I'd think how unfathomable it was that I was able to make the journey, my body unable to move any more, my mind cloudy and weary. But before the thought passed, I would fall asleep in my King's arms, and for the next eighteen hours, it'd be my King and I, husband be damned. While my husband was aware of the toll my illness was taking on me, it was especially during those evenings when he arrived home from work earlier than usual that the magnitude of my disease would hit home for him. Entering the house without any sign of me, he would climb the stairs, observing my strewn clothes littering the hallway, and enter our bedroom, spying me, peaceful and still, with my King. Many hours later when I would awake in my King's embrace, I worried that my husband felt helpless, not only since the illicitness of my relationship with my King would normally occur while my husband was at the office putting in a full day at work, but also because it was my King, not my husband, who provided me with the comfort and support I so desperately desired and needed. I felt like I was being deceptive, even though my fatigue, which was my predominant MS symptom, was very much out in the open.

Soon, as my fatigue became insurmountable, my King began holding me hostage. And because I was now so ill, no matter how hard I tried to resist, I obeyed his beckoned call. I began to lose confidence and my own identity, for without my King, who was I? Now I had truly become one with my King—a symbiotic relationship gone terribly awry. Even though I knew it wouldn't do much good, I considered downgrading to a Queen, but Her Majesty was never my cup of tea. And twins reminded me too much of a horny teenage boy's wet dream. So, after almost a year of living this way, under my King's lock and key, I knew I had to take some serious action. But what price was I willing to pay to escape the stronghold of my King once and for all?

My doctors had tried to free me from the grips of my King—even my family had attempted to intervene—but to no avail. Weekly, I'd cry to my therapist about the predicament I'd found myself in. So the question remained—What would it take for me to find myself free when I was completely powerless over my King and all interventions had thus far failed? I had already experimented with the injectable interferon medications to slow down the MS disease process, as well as monthly intravenous steroids for energy and every pill that had been shown to have some effect on MS lassitude. But because I hadn't been seeing results, I began receiving monthly infusions of a controversial medication. This so-called MS "wonder drug" had had a short and tenuous history and an uncertain future, linked to causing a deadly brain infection. But when my fatigue worsened to the point where I was no longer living an independent life, the decision to begin taking this drug was clear if I was ever to have the chance of escaping my King ... -sized bed, that is. If I were to obtain a crown of my own, I saw this drug as my only chance. I was hopeful and excited to begin treatment, because I needed to believe there was a way out of this mess, a possibility I would be able to live the vast majority of my life independently beyond the control of my King. Because I began experiencing some positive changes after a few infusions— less fatigue, a decrease in pain, and an improvement in spasticity—I truly believed this to be in the cards for me.

Now one year—and fourteen infusion treatments—later, I have yet to receive that elusive crown, the medication not serving as my knight in shining armor. Well, I guess I never believed in fairy tales anyway. While the medication has given me a handful of fatigue-free days, it has not dramatically altered the quality of my life as I had hoped. However, while I still spend the majority of my days with my King, I am no longer his hostage. Even though at times I find myself succumbing to my King's seduction, there is now an understanding between my King and me, a partnership per se, and more often than not, I avail myself of his warm re-energizing embrace. Time has a way of altering perception, and although it has been a struggle to accept my changed reality, in the past year I have made progress coming to grips with my situation. My life has changed considerably in the years since my MS diagnosis, and while I remain optimistic about the new medications and treatments on the horizon, I assume my life may not improve much until a cure for MS is discovered. Yet, because I realize imperfect realities are part of the human condition, I am focused on living my life to the fullest extent possible within the parameters dictated by my disease. I may stumble along the way, but I can rest assured that my King will see me through as I embark on this new phase in my life. Carpe diem.

Anne Anderson

The Operation

Diagnosis

Heart pounds loudly
Fright grips my soul
Doctor tells us "I am an expert
After all.............."
Three pancreatic cancers done weekly
Expert knows it all
Does three surgeries a week
Pounding heart
Drowns out words
Fear grips my in-most being
Not believing words
I remain immobile
Nameless anguish
The door to Hell
Opens widely

Pain Without End

Surgery over
Doctor feels successful
 I drown in pain
Broken glass shards
Stabbing pain
The "I" becomes the pain

Discharge

Time to go home
HMO policy says so
White blood cells elevated
Temperature shoots for the moon
103° of heat
Doctor looks the other way

Home Alone

Pain, stabbing pain
Three days of eternity pass
Wound opens
Hell widens

My View of the Opening

Look down on blood and pus
Flowing onto bed
Recognize pancrease—it is still there
Very sick and weak
Consumed by fear
Wet with blood and pus
Inner life fluids flow dangerously
Frightened but still alive
911 arrives
Finally, breathe deeply

Adjusting to Endless Changes/Losses

Many changes in my body since medical error entered my life

Abilities gone
Former strengths melt to fears of self-assurances

Multiple losses
I can no longer practice my work I so dearly loved
Dependency towers over self-sufficiency
Slightest activities melt away self-sufficiency

What does the future hold for me?
Will my finances be adequate to meet all my mounting necessities?
I see my pharmacist more often than former friends

What road must I take on this journey forced onto me?
What lies around the corner?
Don't really want to know

I can no longer make plans.
Traveling to visit grandchildren overwhelms me
The "what ifs" and other uncertainties win

Friends avoid me to protect themselves from discomfort of human frailty.
They, too, may face vulnerabilities some day

Making Rounds with Dr. Elliot P. Joslin MD

Nurses sit in Nurses' station, weary
From a busy night of caring for youth:
Struggling to live with diabetes.

Dr. Elliott P. Joslin MD enters to begin
Morning rounds. He is smiling and gentle
As nurses dutifully rise to stand.
"Miss La Pointe, please make rounds with
Me this morning," as he reaches for charts.

Rounds begin in a ward occupied by adolescents.
They struggle to live lives with diabetes
And its accompanying vicissitudes of diabetes.

Shared picture of youthful despair; many eyes closed.
At times fear reflected from their deepest self.
Diabetes, Type I … unpredictable and rows of lethargic
Youth lie before us. In the background I look up.
I see the IV hung dutifully and connected to needle-pricked
Hands and arms dripping slowly and methodically.

"Miss La Pointe," Dr. Joslin inquires: "What do you see,
Hear, smell, touch" as we pause by his bedside. Face of
Fifteen year old is pale, skin moist and clammy.
Youth is speechless and appears sleeping soundly.
Far, far away from this world.

Breath fruity to the senses as I bend over, closer. Gently
Touching his moist skin on his arms as tears fall
Upon my crisp white uniform. Pondering to self,
"He is so young."

Dr. Joslin speaks assuredly and ever so carefully injects 1cc
Of regular, life giving insulin into the IV.
IV hangs by his side awaiting its role in this drama.
Young, brown eyes open widely and look about
As he returns to this world and his surroundings.

Surely, I have seen a miracle. Dr. Joslin had a special commitment
To his patients, especially the children. His dedication to
Their care was like no other.

Suzanne Edison

The Arousing: Thunder, Keeping Still: Mountain, Preponderance of the Small

I had forgotten the rope around my ankles
the unseen anchor, noose, we wove

until you called, mother, to confirm
aggressive progressive no cure.

When you asked for my help to die
my ankles burned. I reached for a knife.

I saw white tablets engraved with faulty instructions,

pills rolled in brittled fingers, their beauty halting,
residue: four children the garden gone

to thickets—a lamp blinking red-green-indigo blue.

Weeks straddling fallen
strands of hair, knots of chit chat

mixed with silence—if not me
who would dish out crush up hand over—

who hold the pillow over your face

your eyes, those bindweed seeds of love

Night Court

Demeter charges Persephone with abandonment

Persephone counter-sues with endangerment

Zeus, excessively tan and late for arraignment, has his parental rights revoked

Hades, who pimps his ride with Persephone's hair tied to his antenna
is charged with racketeering, crossing state lines and ordered to perform
community service.

In Family court the judge asks for parting comments

Hades says to Persephone, "I'm sure we will meet again"

and Demeter says, "Over my dead body"

Jen Cross

Excerpted from s^{s}i^{s}t^{e}e^r: a de-ology

(1986)

Dear somebody:

My sister knows I like to write. I make up poems, find words for dreams, so she gives me cloth-covered books with lined empty pages, but those just sit on my bookshelf 'til I have something pretty to put in them. This way that I want to be talking to you out there (*Aren't you somewhere? Couldn't there be somebody?*) shouldn't really go down on paper. Somebody in the house might find it, probably my sister and she would show it to him because we get points, kind of, for betraying each other. I'll leave them somewhere secret. Maybe you'll find them.

I feel like you'll know what I mean. It's kind of like you're already in my head, you already know all the stories, everything that's happened and happening even though I still want to tell you about it. There isn't anybody else. Mom is too much with him. Kimmy and I can't keep each other's secrets anymore. I can't have any friends at school—they all talk to him already, or could, since I don't know which ones he sees in his practice; he has to keep that information confidential. It's the ethical thing to do.

(I don't like to use his name, my stepdad; it's dangerous. You know that already.)

Sometimes I feel like I live on another planet. Like all the other kids at my high school get to go home and eat some kind of snack and do their homework or hang out on the phone until it's dinnertime and their mom makes dinner and they eat with their mom and they get dessert and they watch some TV or their friend comes over in their own car and they go to some other friend's house to hang out and then they come home and go to sleep when they want to or even earlier if they're told to and they get up the next morning right before school and they shower and rinse out their sour mouths and eat cereal and toast and drive to school or catch the bus or their same friend or maybe boyfriend or girlfriend comes to get them and they make it to school just when the bell is ringing for homeroom.

That's not how it is for me, for us, on the planet Kimmy and Mom and I live on.

Last night he got mad because Mom did something wrong in therapy with the people from Boys Town, and we all had to stay at the table after dinner while he talked to her. That afternoon, he had been upstairs with Kimmy a long time after school and I was supposed to watch the door for them, in case Mom came home early. I kept the TV on, of course, so I wouldn't hear them. Unfortunately, that meant I didn't hear mom's car when she actually did come home early—I couldn't believe it. It was just 6:00, and we all had to rush to get dinner made because we thought she would be home closer to 7:30 and he would have time to take me upstairs and Kimmy was supposed to get dinner started during that. I heard the key in the lock and yelled *Hi Mom* so he could get himself to the shower. I told Mom that Kimmy was doing homework.

So, instead of me being in trouble for not getting dinner ready in time, Mom got in trouble because she came home too early and interrupted him with Kimmy, but she didn't know that, of course. She was sad and disappointed. She thought she would be able to come home early and surprise us, then we could all make dinner together and have a good night, but he was dripping and cranky like he always was after he had sex with her, I mean with mom—I never understood why sex would make him so angry and foul. She didn't have time to recognize his mood or get an answer to why he was showering in the middle of the evening because he demanded to know why she said what she said during the therapy group they did that day with abused boys from the group home; you'd think she never had been a therapist on her own for so many years the way he talks to her: like, if she's so bad, why are you in private practice with her? While he was talking to her in the living room, I tried to thaw some hamburger quickly under running water in the sink so I could make spaghetti sauce and I knew he might get mad because we had spaghetti only a few days ago but it was the fastest thing I could get on the table. I fried the meat in the nonstick pan that we have special utensils to clean and stir with, and when it was all thawed and cooked through and brown, I dumped jarred spaghetti sauce on it. I always finish thawing the meat in the pan—he says I'm impatient and don't know how to follow the rules. I broke up the still-frozen pieces with the spatula, pink and icy on the inside while they're brown and cooked and oily on the outside. I made a salad with iceberg lettuce that I tore instead of cut so it didn't rust, and chopped tomatoes and sliced carrots and onion. I started to set the table and when Kimmy finally came downstairs, in the clothes she wore to school, she helped me set the table and took over the sauce and tested the spaghetti. We didn't make eye contact but one of us made some dumb joke about mom or how his dog looked like a fat greasy white sausage and what if we cooked her and she'd be brown and furry on the outside and pink on the inside and that broke the ice and made us laugh quietly while Mom and he get louder. We don't call it arguing. We're lucky our parents don't fight. They just talk. He calls her stupid and unprofessional and wants to know when she's going to deal with her shit.

Kimmy didn't get in trouble for wearing her school clothes to dinner or for leaving her bookbag at the foot of the stairs. My body felt tight and vibrating, kind of tingly but not all the way numb; he wasn't mad at me yet because mom came home early and he couldn't take me upstairs to my room and use his mouth. (I guess I'll have to do it tomorrow, or soon. I wanted to go to chess club tomorrow but he will want me to come home, to him, will call me a slut because I joined chess club because of a boy I like. I am not really learning to play chess. I just learn the names to all the pieces and how they move. The pawn can go forward or back but only one space. The bishop can go diagonally, the knight goes in an L. I like that one a lot. The queen can go anywhere but she's the one that all the other pieces, even the king, are supposed to protect. You win when you take down the queen.)

I put cubes of ice in all the glasses and poured the pop in, then I put the bowls of spaghetti and sauce and salad on the table. Kimmy put down the placemats over the table cloth and folded the napkins to one side of the plates and put the silverware on either side of the plates. I put on serving utensils and the bottles of salad dressing and the can of parmesan cheese. Then Kimmy told them that dinner was ready.

It's hard to digest when he's talking with one of us. Mom's face was still strong when she came to the table. She hadn't cried yet, but he's never done with her until she really understands what she did wrong and cries and is ashamed and says she's sorry. She wore her work clothes, a multicolored jacket from one of the fancy stores in the Old Market, black linen pants and a cream camisole. He was in his house shirt and torn, work-around-the-house pants, and his hair is still wet from the shower, slicked back from his face like it was morning. He served himself some spaghetti, but Kimmy and mom and I waited a minute. Then Kimmy served herself first of the three of us, a little impatient, and then he said to Mom, *Well, go ahead and eat might as well not let this meal go to waste that your girls made for you even though you're full of your shit.* I didn't look at her when she passed the bowls to me because either she'd get in more trouble for duping me into smiling at her or I'd be in trouble for colluding with her illness, her mental difficulty, her shit. (That's what he says we all have: illness to work out. He doesn't have anything to work out; he's done his work already, he says.)

Kimmy and I don't look at each other. The food doesn't have any taste.

(1979)

Dear somebody:

My sister follows me everywhere.

I'm bundled in the blue coat with the canvas outside and the fuzz in the inside and the fuzz all around the hood. My sister's and my hoods were around our faces or down around our necks, hanging loose like animal skins. We wear thick denim Lee jeans, red galoshes. Kimmy follows me, out into the sludge-snowy backyard, behind the wood frame house where mom was reading her cookbooks and dad was going to sleep. It's winter break, and all the friends in my first grade class with Miss Schmidt are away visiting relatives, so I'm daring Kimmy to taste the ice.

We had heard stories about the danger, and dared each other to put our mouths to the oil tank that sat to the side of the house, coated in frost and wet new snow. I want her to go first but she won't. Reaching my face forward, the tank smells like the inside of dad's garden hose, but colder. I touch my tongue to the top of the enormous rusted metal oil tank, just a flick, so I can get the snow and frost off, quick enough that the flesh doesn't catch on the cold metal. Heat rushes through me, and I feel like I've escaped something big. I haven't ever had my tongue stuck to anything metal outside in the winter but I know it could be bad.

Kimmy follows my lead. I knew she could get her tongue stuck. I might not have warned her. I might get a little smug when I see she was stuck. She pulls her head back sharply, then squeals and starts to cry. Suddenly my stomach goes hard and bad; that feeling expands to fill my arms and legs, and my head gets heavy. My sister can't move because the flesh of the inside of her mouth is caught on the metal tank that's on the east side of the house, hidden between our house and the fence that keeps us from the next house over. An old woman lives there who has big fruit trees in the front that flower in spring, and we pick the white bundles of blooms and pink buds for May Day baskets.

This isn't spring. Kimmy's scared and I have to run inside, go in through the back door that opens flat into the back yard. Inside the house are our back stairs and walls lined with shelves and storage. Up the stairs, around the corner, is the kitchen. Where are my mom and dad? The house always feels empty even if we are all there. Child spirits don't fill a house, especially when we are trying to stay out of the way of our parents' too-big sadness. We don't know why they're sad. All we know is the inside silence—silence inside them. We keep outside a lot. *(Those were the Outside years. The Inside years come later.)*

My mother comes out with sharp notes at me and cooing warming notes to my sister. She slowly pours warm tap water over the place where Kimmy's tongue meets the iron. Maybe some of my sister's flesh stays behind. She's crying, hurt and scared, and my mom is mad at me for not warning my sister and my sister is confused: *Did you know? Did you know?* And I'm ashamed: how do you say yes to her face? I try to harden up against the squishy, oozing guilt: *Of course I knew, stupid. Everyone knows!* But I can't say *stupid* in front of mom. We get in trouble for things like that.

I say *I'm sorry, Kimmy.* I want my sister to believe in me.

(1993)

Dear somebody:

Later, after time has shifted off its usual axis (*and even now it isn't back yet, it will never be back*), I learn the skill of rolling time in my mouth alongside his fingers or tongue or maybe penis—by now there is a *he,* a *his.* By now, there is a single un-antecedent-able pronoun. It comes to be how I divide the people in my world, my friends here at college. If you know me at all, you know who he is.

Before I left for college, we know about each other, she and I: *we know about each other,* like a wife and a lover, like two girlfriends a man has—or like sisters who have been separated, isolated, and suddenly re-introduced to each other.

There are things to explain to you, I guess: How we used to be one another's touchstones for years, the place where each turned to check: *if she's there everything is ok. I'm ok.* We were each other's steady point and gumption, each other's mouths and hearts. She tasted things through me, would wait for me to put something new onto my tongue first and wait to read my face before she would eat it herself: *if I didn't like it she wouldn't touch it.* (I wasn't there to taste, to test, the first time my stepdad came for her.)

We were sisters in the truest, fairy tale sense: kindred in blood heart and utterly opposite in the world. Her social and golden, me darker, more likely to be found alone, even back in the land of Before.

But I meant to tell you a scene from Later: We are on the futon bed on the floor in the basement. Kimmy and I are flat on our backs and naked and pale and lithe and long-haired, and we are deeply lovely—our faces similar enough that we are mistaken for twins and yet when I look at her face and then mine in a mirror I can't understand anywhere in my bones how people could think someone so pretty looks like me. Her face is a slope of joy. She has bright eyes and her hair is lighter than mine, finer and wavy—it curls sometimes all on its own. Her eyebrows are lighter, her nose more buttony, her face more oval, less square, all of her finer-featured.

We have our legs and arms in the air like we are dancing. We are dancing a horizontal can-can, we are laughing and her laugh sounds like power and freedom to me like we can control anything we want, we are alone in this laughter and the watcher part of me wants him to know that. He is naked too and he has his small video camera in his hands, over his eyes and he films our giggling dancing naked faces, our bouncing legs. He tries to tell us what to do. My sister and I hold hands and don't listen.

(Just recently, when I was having sex with three friends in college, the woman I am in love with and two male friends I care for quite a bit, the woman I am in love with grabbed my hand at one point. This sex, all the ministrations and orchestrations came together so we could touch each other, so we could have our own kind of sex separate from the young men, but maybe I had been too nervous not to have men there or we just really wanted to do everything there was to do. She took my hand and I felt fragmented, like I was there in bed with my sister again, except now there were men over each of us instead of just one of us at a time. And even though these men are kind and my good friends, I felt that indelible nausea and rage on both of our behalves and I wanted only to get our friends out of us and onto each other so we could be alone, she and I, and safe.)

Later he filmed other things, us doing other things. I don't want to tell you that yet. I don't know what happened to the video tape.

(2009)

Dear somebody:

This is what my story contains: this wreckage that is all of our wreckage, the fragmentary remembering that is never more than anyone else's remembering but feels like less, necessarily, because of the shroud trauma and loss cast over every indecent obelisk of that reckoning: an ornate crimson tinting, veiling the sharp delineated carve and curvature of breath—

The way trauma is constantly whispering in my inside ear, asking *Really? Are you sure? Are you sure? Are you sure?* like static, that haze freezing the smooth flow of my pen as soon as I drop my hand to the page and begin to write. Static, the way a radio tuning goes cloudy sometimes once you remove the antenna your body provides when you pull your hand away and expect the music to keep on flowing smoothly on its own

This metaphor could extend indefinitely, remix with others, entwine, commingle, shadow, stave off: but what's there is this girl holding a stepfather's balls in her one hand while his tiny, foreshortened penis   shoves   rocks   pushes in and out of her mouth. The clouds shroud my shoulders as I write, the way her mouth clouded, too, eventually, filmy and white, and this was the living room couch and she was as worried as he was of getting caught—*getting caught*—by her mother, his wife, the innkeeper, who was in the kitchen in the bathroom in the office, who was keeping to herself after a day of his constant monitoring at the private practice office they shared.

The one with the him on the couch, she's 16 or 17 or 18 or 19 or 20, this could have been any of those ages, I won't risk the static return by venturing to determine which one it was exactly. Her limbs might have looked long and coltish and adult and her mouth would taste clotted and congealed and corpulent, and this moment lives in nobody's memory of her except his and her own because who else can contain this kind of history? The parents and lovers who have heard the stories are longing to be rid of them, to shed their ears of the words as soon as they're spoken, as soon as the breath around each component syllable has cooled and I write because I don't want him to be the one still who knows me best in the world, most intimately, who knows all of my most fragmentary and unspeakable secrets.

Vomit up what I've told you, if you like. I'd like to. I think it's the only reason I used to drink to such excess—heaving isn't something my body does on command. If you can do it, though, then we can all bear witness to the marshaled splatters, the detailed reserves, our history finally visible for all to see.

Jennifer Stevenson

What They Carry

> They carried all they could bear, and then some, including a silent
> awe for the terrible power of the things they carried.
>
> Tim O'Brien, *The Things They Carried*

Into the oncology unit at Stanford hospital the patients brought all kinds of things to make their stay more comfortable, more like home. They brought carefully cleaned pillows and blankets. They brought pajamas and other comfortable clothes.

Most of them did not bring many white blood cells.

Some of them had to wear masks if they felt up to leaving their rooms; what looked like gas masks from the 50s. I saw one of my patients, a seventy-year-old vibrant woman—who recently went to the doctor due to fatigue and came out with a diagnosis of leukemia—sitting in the posh Stanford hospital lobby listening to classical music wearing her big mask, her face obscured, and she herself tucked between her big white-haired husband and her forty-year-old daughter, Paulette. All mask, she sheepishly waved to me. She carried her one favorite pink robe that made her look like a girl.

The nurses carried different things from the patients: stethoscopes and scissors, tape in small fanny packs attached to their waist, saline flushes and medications. Some of them carried pictures of their family to remind them of how lucky they were and why some days they did their job. They carried the burden of student nurses or new nurses who usually needed more help than they could provide. They also endured an understanding that sometimes no matter how hard they pushed on the residents or attendings they had trouble getting their patients' needs met. They buried the sadness that came with each death just as much as they celebrated the patients who walked out carrying their own things home.

As a student nurse, I carried a fearful curiosity. Behind her door, Giselle, my seventy-year-old patient in the pink fleece robe, taped a picture of my cat to the window.

How is Chloe the cat today? she would ask in her lilting Belgian accent. And then we would talk of things so light they floated away through the cracks of the door.

Giselle carried the fear that her husband could not care for himself if she were to die. He was old and diabetic and he carried her always in his eyes. How did you get this sweet man to propose? I teased one day.

No, no, her husband brushed away my playfulness with his cane, I was the lucky one. Forty-five years of marriage. You see that ring; that ring came from my grand-mother—and so Giselle carried on a family tradition represented by a shiny silver band that came from Belgium. Giselle had carried three babies in her life and the eldest, Paulette, was there at the hospital all of the time. She stayed at a residence for family members across the street where she cooked for her father, helped him manage his diabetes, and cooked things that her mother might eat. Giselle carried a sense of fullness that made her nauseous, like being pregnant, she yelled with a forced grin.

Paulette carried the worry of her mother's illness, acute lymphocytic leukemia, and her father's fragile health; she carried the guilt she felt at being away from her own family, the husband she adored and her two girls.

We all carried the weight of knowledge or a lack of it: the daily blood counts, the fevers, the subtle signs of infection. Ideas about fairness and love and things ending too soon.

A widow and a feisty special education teacher, Ms. Hill, was another patient I carried. Her room was filled with paper cards of stick people with round heads that said: Get Better SOON!! Each day I checked her neuro status with the typical questions: what day is it ... what year? Then I decided to change my questions since patients often memorize the information you ask of them over and over again. So I brilliantly asked her: what holiday did we just have. She paused. Then quietly whis-pered, Christmas. With a painful insight, she longingly sighed, I've missed all the best ones this year.

I looked at the dates on the cards more carefully—they were sent in late September; it was winter now. The cards themselves were yellowing around the edges.

Ms. Hill carried an inner drive to see her grandchildren. So even though she had lost all of her hair, begun losing her vision and the ability to smell, she insisted on the three times daily nasal lavage for her now growing sinus fungal infection. Even though it made her vomit and she could barely hold anything down anyway, Ms. Hill carried a dignity with her. Swollen-eyed, she demanded to be bathed a certain way and even though some of the nurse's aides found her caustic, I found that following her directions as she asked made her quite pleasant. As I left her room week after week, I carried the concern that her mental status was changing; she believed something was in her mouth, something large and metal.

One day I left her room, swallowed my fear, and listened to the intern's report on Ms. Hill during rounds. The intern said nothing about her mental status so I looked at the attending and said: there is something else here. He waited. I explained that it wasn't just a metal taste that sometimes comes from chemo treatments but the experience of something in her throat and mouth—something metal—she was sure there was a foreign object inside her mouth. The attending blinked and looked at his intern. Why haven't you ordered a CT scan? The intern glared at me.

I am sure the intern carried his own fears and a workload so intense that he was almost bent over. I carried the anger I felt as one of the experienced nurses gave me a talking to afterward—never embarrass an intern in front of his attending. I protested, I thought we were a team.

Not exactly, she told me.

Later that week, as I carried Ms. Hill's lavage materials out of the room, I heard another team rounding about her case, their words added to the things I carried: there's no more we can do. Who wants to tell Ms. Hill she's going to hospice? The attending looked around the small group of interns who found something fascinating about the ugly hospital carpet. I put those words deep into my heart where the now sightless Ms. Hill wouldn't see them and returned to her room.

Where have you been? she tried to yell. We have to do this three times a day so I can get out of here. And so for an hour I used a 60 ml syringe filled with an anti-fungal and saline water while Ms. O'Brien inhaled each syringe full deep into her sinuses, held it as long as she could until it exploded out of her nose and her mouth. We kept another container for emesis. Do you want to stop and rest? NO! she retorted. Dinnertime is almost here and I have to eat the whole thing. I have to. So we continued: five times in each nare, both of us covered in water and blood and mucous. We'll keep going, Ms. Hill said. Okay, I replied as she vomited up her dinner. I wondered who outside the door would carry the news that Ms. Hill did not want to hear.

As I left her room, I noticed the intern on call that night carried the phone from which she learned something that caused her to grab onto a desk. It was the pathologist, telling her that a seventeen-year-old patient had aspergillus in her lungs. She let out a sad sigh while she mouthed the name of the fungus that we both knew would end the girl's life.

The family members carried in pictures of themselves, meals that were cooked and not laden with bacteria. They brought child-like things, like stuffed animals. The patients always had clocks and calendars. Every door was the same, a calming mild brown wood slab behind which the patients kept all of their things they were allowed.

That last night of my rotation I went home, carrying my dirty scrubs and more knowledge than I felt I could handle.

Carol Howard-Wooten

25 Years
Living with Stroke

Do Not Edit

Just Listen

I'll play by
My rules today
Stop trying to fit in

Shuffling the pages of poems
Passed around the table
Finding the one you are reading
Is hard.

I try anyway
I want to look smart
I really want you to slow down
I need space between all the words

Understanding the words flying around my head
Impossible
It ain't happening
I listen anyway.

My nervous system jangles, shakes, quivers
Like fear. Or cold.
I ignore it. Pretend I'm with you. Try to fit in.

I listen in my way

Your words fly around my head like airplanes
There is a place inside they once landed
Lined up
Made sense

Your words fly around my head like airplanes
This control tower needs them
To land
Slowly

Limitations: You know what it's like to live with them when you have them

I want our group of stroke survivors
To slash pumpkins on the lawn
And have someone film us.

Maybe then Dr. Tom
Who was a surgeon
Now, paralyzed on one side
Would dare join us
Rather than slash his wrist again.

Insistent

2:25 The white Westclox
I bought for my mother

Dead One Year
(One Year Dead)

· 2:30 AM
June 28, 2010

I wear her nightgown
Sleep on her sheets

The comfort here
surprises me
I spent years
not being
HER

Home Hospice

For three months my father lay dying
The hospital bed filled the living room.

Each morning my mother insisted
Luz weigh him before breakfast.

"Eighty-eight pounds"
whispered Luz.

"He's dying mother. Let him eat!"
There. I said it.

The number mattered more than a warm egg.
I knew she thought she was keeping him alive.

Terri Pauser Wolf

The Stories Remain

The following stories are random samples from a longer memoir about life as an oncology nurse.

The Scribe

Once my fingers were smeared with ink, a writer's blood. The ink is long washed off my hands. Now my stories are written in red in the lifeblood of those looking to ease their suffering. They come with tumors and fevers, broken bones, a twitch, and they want medicine to fix it. There is no pill in any pharmacy in this town that can change their stories. They are living the stories. They are the stories. This is the scribe I want to be—a nurse, a witness to the life stories of others. A chance to tell the world they count, they're important. They exist.

Human Connection

It's our human connection that counts, that remains with me always. All the stuff of my medical world disappears: the syringe wrappers incinerated, the drugs metabolized, the orders archived in the electronic medical records system. We move on to the next person in line with more hope, more treatments, but the stories remain. They crawl inside me, and I will take them with me and share them with you, so you may know these survivors or the departed.

Paper Stories

Several times a day, I tear white wrinkled paper from the adult-sized exam room table and toss it in the trash, readying this drab space for the next patient. Underneath that ball of paper rests the packaging from medical supplies that I had opened throughout the day. This wastebasket holds the sediment of the day, its layers giving clues to the people who had come through the door.

Someone poking through this trash would just see garbage as they uncovered layers of paper balls, blood drawing supplies, medication information, and crumpled tissues. Each stratum reveals a piece of the story of children and cancer.

The last person to sit on the table was a pre-teen in pink sweatshirt and pants, hugging her Beanie Baby horse, her hairless head gleaming under the fluorescent light. She clasped her hands over her face in frustration that her not feeling well, not eating, her pale skin was an automatic reservation to a hospital bed. She had hoped as she and her mom made the seventy-mile journey that the doctor would have some magic brew in his black bag, a tonic that would give back her teen-hood, but that wouldn't happen today. Soon she'd be lying on a mechanical bed fitted with sheets starched as much as the paper, behind special doors where, in each room, a special filter hummed as it scrubbed the air of bacteria and fungus and microbes that could kill her.

She wasn't the only one to sit on the crinkly paper and hear bad news. Another heard about an advancing brain tumor—one sending out shoots and roots into a five-year-old's head. His young parents were launching a business, just hanging on and then this—this intrusion. The three of them—mom, dad and son—sit on the exam table, the paper splitting beneath them, as they shift around trying to find a comfortable position to hear the news. Grandpa leans against the counter with arms folded. He's the Chemo Daddy to his grandson when mom and dad must show up for work. His life will be different now, too, as two doctors with paper on clipboards make notes, take notes, and talk about this unexpected development in a tumor that had already been treated.

The family leaves the room and takes their son to the infusion room where I'll meet them after opening boxes of chemotherapy drugs that the doctor wants given. Soon a blue pump rhythmically squirts new chemo into his vein, the watery bag holding hope for a sixth year. He's unaware of the change and is eager to get out the puzzle. He and his mom sit in little chairs at the round kindergarten-size table and start interlocking pieces. A large dinosaur image appears from the cardboard—the one mom wants to eat away the tumor. She fidgets with the pieces, wondering how it will all fit together. She laughs with her son as if the world is the same and this is the most normal thing to do—spend a day playing with your son, her back to the pump pushing in yet another possibility.

The numbers on the pump turn with new digits coming across the screen. I dream: Wouldn't it be grand if there was a bar to pull like a Las Vegas slot machine where you could go for the win—the life jackpot—the clean MRI—where bells and whistles would ring, and you could hear the excited call from the floor manager and get your life back? As I look at these numbers, what is put into the slot, I'm not seeing the three bars. Like in Las Vegas casinos, a few win and the rest go away with empty pockets. In this child's case and type of tumor, the statistics are with the house. One day his parents will exit this hospital emptied of their dreamed-of life.

I leave this mother-son team as another child needs attention. The little girl moves her boated six-year-old body from her kid-sized wheelchair to the exam table and nearly blends in with the white paper background. She is in white sweatpants and a white sweatshirt with skin so pale it's as if all of her red blood cells have escaped. Steroids puff her cheeks and slap on a ruddy stain. She's in agony, groaning and irritable.

Her mother, sitting on a short stool, leans on the edge of the exam table, her hand rubbing her daughter's leg, wanting it to be consoling. The crinkly white paper turns translucent where her mother-tears drop. Her shoulders hunched, she exclaims, "I don't know what to do!" How could she know? Dr. Spock never wrote a chapter for this, the child dying from brain cancer.

A bed is ready in the hospital and her daughter is whisked off the table and wheeled to the 7th floor for pain control and to give mom a break. I step back into the empty room and see her imprint, the crinkles where she lay. I tear off the paper, crumple it and put it in the trash, knowing I will do it again and again during this day, building up the layers.

After 5 AM when the clinic doors lock, a janitorial crew will sweep through and empty these paper balls, wipe down the tables, and mop the floor, not knowing the mess they're really cleaning up. They'll take the trash away to a distant plant where the paper will be incinerated, vaporizing the stories. My pen will become my personal janitor, the opportunity to use words to mop up this misery.

What Do You Fear?

I fear making a mistake. Words I can erase. I can play with them before releasing them. I can't take back the wrong dose already pushed into the vein by a pulsing IV. I can't get it back. I can't stop the omission of not remembering how to deal with your heart—stopped. How much epinephrine and when?

I fear making a mistake that might cost you your life or your limb, as I rush to please everyone and be timely. I might assume or misread the label. The line is incredibly slim, and it's taut as airline cable. The recoil from its snap can be deadly.

Oh, please, guide my hands, my eyes that I treat you perfectly, that you get the medicine you need in the right way at the right times and in the right amount.

My fear is measured in milligrams and micrograms.

What is that Smell?

They never told me about this smell. A dozen nursing professors, hours of clinical time at hospitals and clinics, and one smell that you're not supposed to know.

It's 3 AM. I'm on the 7th floor of the medical center in teal scrubs that I've only worn once before, my white cross-trainer shoes without a stain. I walk into ICU Room 3 and into a spot by the side-rail nearest his head to begin my start of shift assessment. I see three IV poles to my left and a TV monitor above my head. Each ole holds two bags of fluids and tubes that connect to powerful medicine going into his body at different junctures. A tangle of latex-free medical spaghetti rests by his right ear, the tubes out of control, like his condition.

He lies still in bed, then restless, and then quiet—typical for a brain injury, I'm told. Scary for day two on the job, finding out what they didn't tell me in nursing school, especially about the smell that I can't quite figure out—the one you're not supposed to know.

I look over his large-for-his-age, thirteen-year-old body. His midsection is wrapped in a diaper, his neck in a spinal collar. His left leg wears a cast, the only obvious wound of being distracted while on a skateboard, looking back at friends and feeling the impact of the car. During report before the shift started, the day nurse started out with, "Kid verses car." She continued with the story: Local paramedics scooped his battered body from the small-town street and deposited him into a medical helicopter for a flight to this large medical center. Once in the trauma center specialists intervened in stopping and sopping up the seeping and gushing fluids. They inserted "lines" all over his body, drilled into and put the cast on the left leg, which now weighs thirty pounds more. He got an admission ticket to the ICU where a tube and machine breathes for him, and several more tubes and machines give him medicine. He doesn't speak. His eyes stare blankly.

The novice new-grad nurse, I get to collect data: heart rate, respirations, temperature, drug titration rates, neurological signs, urine input and output. As I move closer for my data collection, unwashed body odors come from inside his spinal collar. I smell the starch of his sheets and there is one odor—a little fruity, apricot with a must that moves by me from time to time. I can't figure out the source.

My supervising nurse, a twenty-year veteran who is here to show me what they didn't teach in school, points to the damp gauze taped under his nose and both ears. He tells me to change them. I fold gauze squares in half and find tape to secure them. As I peel off the old, saturated gauze, the odor surrounds me, and I'm curious. "What is this fluid?" I ask.

"Cerebral spinal fluid," smirks the nurse.

I look at the boy's mother on the other side of the bed awkwardly curled into a chair, sleeping. I think about my similar aged children safe at home. Even in my beginner's place, I know this is something you should never smell or see—amber liquid draining from this boy's Humpty Dumpty crack. We couldn't put him back together again.

Claire Badaracco

The Middle Surgeon

The Hospice worker said my feeling was common among caregivers, to be expected, that we were riding on an accelerating carousel without Kaliope, spinning at such a rate it was impossible to slow down. My eighty-five-year-old mother had been a lab technologist with two years of university pre-med training before marrying, so blood chemistry was more or less a household word when a routine medical check up caught the high red cell count and the doctor diagnosed Polycythemia Vera, the overproduction of red blood cells. The medical literature admitted "insufficient research exists" to offer an explanation for the actual "cause," asserting the condition occurred mainly in beef-eating men in their fifties and sixties, that it was unheard of in women or in the elderly. When my dainty 5'2" mother was diagnosed, she was vigorous, sharp-minded, independent. The clinical literature said she had two years without treatment, and an indefinite time with routine phlebotomies to manage the skyrocketing red cell count and a low dose chemotherapy pill to reduce the number of sticky platelets. The side effects of chemotherapy in a pill form, even a child's dose—dizziness, weakness, insomnia, loss of appetite, thirst—made the most ordinary of bodily functions seem a gift out of time. During the last fourteen months of her life when I was her primary caregiver, I split many pills and poured the powder from the capsules, being careful not to breathe in anything. I'd think about what science historians called "medicalizing" women, what had occurred in the mid-nineteenth century, when poisons were given to women by doctor-preachers, who not only administered the "heroic cures" as medicine but at the same time preached bedside sermons such as "The Adaptation of our Condition to our Peculiar Wants." It was Oliver Wendell Holmes, lecturing to the all-male class at Harvard Medical School in his farewell address, who said, "Science is the topography of ignorance." A century and a half later, here I stood giving my mother poisons—chemo, warfarin—what we both knew would not heal but would prolong her life, and involve more suffering. What does "quality of life" mean for the frail elderly? Each caregiver is forced to rethink the meaning of these words, for their own well being during the end stage of a loved one's disease.

So my once vigorous, still elegant and beautiful mother joined the many other patients in the Blood Disorders and Hematology Clinic of a leading medical center staffed by twenty highly trained physicians. Patients filled the waiting room, all ages and ethnicities, white and black, pregnant young mothers, teenagers and aged great grandmothers, the rail thin and the fat and ruddy. Clearly, disorders of the blood were an equal opportunity disease, and while the medical science literature had been inadequate about polycythemia vera, there were innumerable variations on cancers of the blood, as it seemed white and red cells could mutate and replicate in ways science could not yet explain. My mother repeatedly asked, "Did they know anyone else with this?" Was she an anomaly? Because of privacy laws the Center could not disclose the names of others in the Clinic with the "rare" disease, even as they all sat in the same waiting room for hours, talking and swapping tales about their respective and various illnesses and how they coped, and my mother continued to search for others who had the Latinate disorder, just someone to talk to about this turn of events, a lethal surprise after a long and healthy life. The way in which disease isolates is spiritual, compounded by the "privacy" laws intended to protect, yet add to a patient's desolation.

After the first diagnosis, the simplest of internet searches revealed several Disease Associations for those with low (but not high) red blood cell counts, low but not high white cell counts, and the "very common" leukemia (or lymphoma) which can be one end-stage result from polycythemia vera. But not in every case was this so, nor was there any discussion of how the disease would mimic diabetes in constricting the blood flow in leg vessels and arteries that would cause gangrene and lead to leg amputation, followed by relentless phantom pain.

In my mother's case, the routine phlebotomies, the letting of blood—another practice out of the history of medicine that had been unchanged except leeches were no longer applied—had to be matched with the intake of saline, or fatal dehydration would occur, and these were administered by nurses in the cancer ward of the clinic lined with beds, and recliner chairs where patients spent many hours hooked up, or leukemia patients weakened by chemotherapy came for their vitamin B12 shots. Her heart rate shot up to 99 during these visits. Though her face and demeanor remained calm, there was no question all this was frightening. In the clinical treatment, the finest nurse we encountered was a man—finest in the sense of his ability to hit the vein the first time, take the blood without bruising the frail arm and paper thin veins, but also in the larger sense of his compassion that was deeply intuitive and went beyond words, to be on the same spiritual level with the patient. He had nursed his own wife through cancer, and her death had left him with children to raise, and so in time he remarried to a widow also left with children, and he had gone on to get his nursing degree, to put food on the table for his double-sized brood. It is not only a medical education, but an educated spiritual understanding by physicians or nurses that they, too, could be the ones attached to that tube, that matter to patients.

A gout-like pain in her toe took two years to develop over the whole foot and leg, and it progressed slowly, with a number of stages. A trip to the podiatrist to cut nails led to a massive swelling and inflammation of her foot, and the closest to a hysterical reaction from her general practice physician who had first diagnosed the condition, provoking a diatribe condemning all and every podiatrist as if they were an antichrist and witchdoctor combined. As a general practice physician, he was a highly competent clinician, usually cool as a cucumber. His hysteria was oddly comforting to us because he was so over the top, and my mother and I giggled like conspiratorial schoolgirls after he exited the examining room, telling my mother to put on her socks and shoes while he consulted his thick volumes of prescription medicines.

The foot swelling and leg edema raised the worries of deep vein thrombosis, more clots that could move up the leg to the heart or brain, and so the hematology specialists sent her to vascular specialists who were surgeons, whose first course of action is to send the patient to radiology for a blood vessel scan. Deeply suspicious of being injected with dye and having a flexible line thread from the groin to the heart in order to detect a blood clot, especially when the dye could be fatal, or the line could disrupt the clot and send it directly to the heart or brain, my mother and I went deep into the windowless interior corridors of the hospital to seek out and find the radiologist on rounds who would have been doing the scan. My mother was limping and supporting herself on her cane. I pretended not to see the people in their last days in the beds lining the radiology ward, all the while my stomach clenched like a fist, stifling the cry "RUN!" We were of a mutual mind that the less medical intervention the better. There should be no elaborate blood vessel scans that required anything inserted in the groin and funneled up arteries to the heart, nothing involving dyes that could sabotage the body and in "rare" cases cause death. Is medical risk factored into care for the elderly who are facing the end ? Is there an underlying ethos in geriatrics that position the high risk test in such a way that the risk is explained away, given that the chances are a quick versus a long drawn out death? My mother was brave, outspoken, assertive, using not only her training but her reading in medicine over the years: yet within she was deeply anxious, aggravating the condition, as more and more tests were prescribed and she was shuttled from one specialist to another to treat the proliferating blood cells. When we were going through these events and days at 250 mph, she never complained and never cried. There was simply no time, only acceptance of suffering punctuated by the high points of each day that consisted of the little things, birds feeding outside the window, the "masseuse" from Hospice who was a retired nun, who brought great smelling creams for her paper thin skin and a bundle of positive thinking about the possibility for tomorrow, leaving with the promise that she would come again in a week. Another care giver who was always in a good mood wore something that sparkled, or sports team logos that engaged her patient in a discussion of an upcoming game involving uproarious crowds and happy contests of the fittest, and alternative reality.

The hospital nurse on duty when my mother and I sought out the radiologist on rounds clearly indicated that she saw the two of us as trouble-makers, because modern medicine requires a passive patient just as it did in the era of Dr. Walter Channing and Sophia Peabody Hawthorne, when it took an unthinkably compliant victim to swallow arsenic or mercury, or breathe ether during labor. The nurse on the radiology ward ushered us to a curtained-off area where we were urged to relax and lower our voices.

Then the radiologist arrived—and he agreed with my mother! Death was indeed a side effect of the test, and he thought also that the risk was too great for a frail woman in her late eighties. And yes, there would be pain involved in the test of course, but he could take care of that with anesthesia—but of course that would entail yet another level of risk. My mother's resistance to the game of double jeopardy was, in the long run, held dear as a grudge by the young female vascular surgeon in the ten-man vascular specialist group practice, who had completed her residency two years before ordering the vein scan. "Well, if you do not want the screening, then we cannot help you further," she sniffed. We left the hospital radiology department full of the dying and the threat of impending or risk of death, and stopped for ice cream on the way back home, our spirits buoyed by Mother's resistance and sharp-minded assertiveness and her ability to talk sense to the highly trained radiologist. She knew her days were numbered, but she had her dignity, and this turned out to be a good day after all.

As her primary caregiver, a humanities major, now a professor, I had associated gangrene with Walt Whitman, the Civil War wounded, something long ago that belonged to battlefields where surgeons had to amputate limbs of soldiers without anesthesia. That was then and this was now. I took her from one doctor to another to examine the foot, and spent long hours in waiting rooms, where we watched as patients with bandaged lower limbs struggled on crutches or sat in wheelchairs, all of them amputees, most visibly and deeply depressed.

When the next surgeon in the practice saw her condition, he gave her the option of amputation of the lower leg above the ankle. When he spoke he did not look at her face, but only at the leg and at me. He acted as if she were not in the room. Coyly nudging my elbow, as if he and I were the co-owners of a shaggy pet, he said, "I could just put her to sleep." His clinical manner stiffened my mother's resistance to any limb loss. Of course he knew the trouble and suffering that lay ahead, for he had seen it many times. He was a specialist in mobility disorders among the elderly. I took her home to suffer as the gangrene spread from one toe to five, then over the whole foot. Gangrene is not literary, I learned the smell of it, and saw what is meant by excruciating pain, for which doctors prescribed hydrocodone, a mix of Tylenol and codeine, and plenty of it.

Seeking a third opinion, we went back, this time to the senior surgeon in the practice, whose attitude and mode of communication represented reasoned compassion, and he offered what Buddhists would call The Middle Way. He said, "arrest the spread of the gangrene" by wrapping the leg in a powerful red antibacterial agent, and "let the gangrene take her" when the time came—but call him immediately when the inflammation began to move up her leg.

The Hospice worker had just left her home after asking me how I felt if my mother died there at home in about three weeks, when I saw the red begin to spread up her leg and made the call to the Middle Way surgeon, who was away on vacation at the time. The fourth surgeon, the youngest in the practice and on call when I phoned on a Saturday said "get here before 8 AM on Monday." Our home health aide came at 6 AM, and wrapping her arms around my mother, lifted her into a wheelchair, then gingerly into the car. Mother was still strong enough to assist and pulled with her arms. Hair grown long during illness was braided into one tail. Wearing a blue beret that matched her eyes, with her favorite pink plaid mohair blanket over her knees, she seemed as poised as a well dressed child going to a party. The aide hopped in the back seat while I drove, white-knuckled, back to the surgeon's.

When we got to the office, he was blunt, a frank style that was the most effective, telling her that she had three days to live, that the choice was hers, and that the leg was already dead but still attached. The three of us sat looking at the black, diseased leg, talking as if it were a stranger, not part of her body at all. I sat off to the side so my presence would not disturb their conversation, so he could ask her directly, "What do you want to do? Amputate the leg above the knee or go into the hospital hospice and die?—you have less than three days to live, and don't even think about going back home, because it is not a possibility." As a doctor he would not release her, but only send her across the street to the hospital, for surgery or hospice. The choice to lose a limb was what she had dreaded all along, saying she was prepared to die rather than to let them cut off her leg. I did not want to make this decision for her, and she could make this end of life decision herself.

What would I do in a similar circumstance? What would you do? Given the option to lose a limb high above the knee, be confined to a nursing home, bedridden, for the rest of her days, or to decide to die in three days? Which choices are the right ones to make at such a time? I certainly did not know, nor did I have any feelings of certainty, only that she was the right one to make the choice, to sign the papers, and I was the one called to support her choice, and just be there with her while she decided what to do, about whether it was better to die or to live and suffer longer. Were we Buddhists instead of Christians, would we have chosen the Middle Way, the option suggested by the middle surgeon, the senior partner in the practice, and let nature take its course? Is prolonging suffering through surgery and pharmaceutical life-support preserving life's "quality," or does it just prolong the natural process of dying, and along with that, suffering?

She chose life: had the leg amputated high above the knee, and survived the surgery, to be confined the rest of her days to a skilled nursing care facility, wheel-chair bound, and then bedridden for about a year. But the nerves remembered the gangrene, and the pain in the lost leg continued every day. Frail and grieving for all the losses—a husband, a son, a leg—she still reached for the empty space in the bed, where her leg would have been ... saying "my foot hurts," still being given the same dose of hydrocodone every four hours as when the diseased leg was attached to her boney frame. Doctors know as little about phantom pain as they do about rare blood disorders. Obviously, it is the nerve endings in the leg that still register the pain, but there must be more to it—the mind remembers the body that was there. The pain remembered is as real as the pain once felt.

Which surgeon was correct? The first one who offered blithely to euthanize her? Everyone knows many a truth lies in jest. Inept as his bedside manner was, he knew the grim prognosis and what suffering lay ahead. The Middle surgeon and senior partner offered a natural death by doing nothing except arresting the gangrene until the time for palliative care. The youngest doctor, with the least experience who worked the weekend call and early Monday morning shift, offered her the moral choice when the time came. But faced with going to the grave sooner without a leg, or later after prolonged suffering, she chose life. I supported her choice, but continued to wonder about the state of scientific knowledge and the blurring of the boundaries between mind and body in medicine, and the vast unknown areas of medical science.

Many physicians and scientists continue to think of Mind-Body medicine as "Alternative," and the very word "phantom" suggests the pain is not real, but "in her head." But locating the pain is as difficult as assigning geography to heaven. Where is it, exactly? Mind-body medicine is integral to the choices everyone makes everyday about preserving and protecting their own health. For the millions of Americans who have stood and will stand by their parents as caregivers, who know every pebble in a road through hell paved with good intentions, how doctors communicate to patients about their end-stage choices is a profoundly complex moral act, and how they communicate determines outcomes. The very essence of life's "quality" is a patient's right to make decisions, even to the end.

Joan Baranow

32 Weeks

There in his isolette he slept
bunched up, like a baguette
warm under the light. The nurse
thought I wanted to hold him,
this soft loaf, I did not, I wished
only to gaze, to let him sleep
in his fetal dream,
but she pulled him out anyway,
looping tubes through the portals
to put him in my arms.
He weighed less than the blanket,
less than a rag doll or cat,
I feared I might drop him
for lightness, a cloth napkin
slipped from my lap. Up close
I saw his pinched forehead,
one eye smaller than the other,
grumpy and anxious.
When he awoke, his mouth crumpled
into weak, fierce cries.
Please, I said, put him back,
so she slid him onto the tray,
adjusted the c-pap, and he curled up
and calmed himself from within.
All he had to do was breathe
and that was enough.

Prescription

Eat a whole mango, its bitter skin
and drippy pulp through to its hairy seed.
Relish the time it takes to pick your teeth
standing on your back porch
watching the dogs run.
By then another hour will have passed.

Feed the dogs. Give Toby her thyroid pill.
Don't assume Robbie is sad.
Don't assume anything.

Plan a trip through the Slavic countries,
the ones with dusky histories and bright,
peppery names. Stay a while in Romania.
I've never been there so you'll need to
take notes. Imagine how great grandma
Freedman lived before the papers came.
Make a packing list of everything
you'll need. You've got grandpa's face,
how he could grin through the worst.

How's the mango tasting? Hold a piece
of its leathery skin under your tongue.
Or spit it out. Who cares? I'm not looking.

Did you get dressed this morning? Go to Walmart
and buy the biggest air mattress on the shelf,
hell, buy a pool too with a filter and cover
and gadgets and picture instructions.
It should take at least three days
just to unfold its sleek vinyl walls.
Then you get to watch your dogs jump in.
Nothing is as happy as a happy dog.

We're all coming to visit. I heard your septic tank
is fixed. Show off your coin collection, your rare books.
We won't go till you tell each story.
Snow's falling already?
That's what Ohio's like, you know that by now.
By March the driveway's full of mung
and the sun's got a permanent film as bad as Plexiglas.
Who wouldn't feel crappy peeling plastic wrap
from another instant dinner? Call me.
We'll laugh at the stupid things Dad did.
We'll forgive each other.

Don't go yet. The world's too screwy without you.
Come see these blue dragonflies touch down
on beach grass. Remember you took me up
in that 2-seater plane? And the alarm went off?
Jesus! That's all I have to say about that.
I'm sending a U-haul to pick up all your dumb
firearms. Get the leash. Toby and Robbie
are licking your shins, ready for a walk.
Take up with a pastry chef. Become a lepidopterist.

Meadow

In this dream you are finally
as light as they said

you would be, before
the body and the birth.

You can see where the hill
has lifted itself

like a breath, where
the last tree has let go its leaves.

And you go there.

David Watts

After Long Silence, Running into my Ex at a Family Gathering

It was not about sorrow,
though a newspaper did blow
across a darkened road,

and we did get helplessly lost
on the way to the Bat Mitzvah.
Sorrow would have been easier

than its recovery,
and that stone-hard certainty
that loss is the end of the sentence.

This was the fragile cellophane
between decorum
and a long swan dive into

the volcano. This
was the song held back,
the coiled spring, tense

and unforgiving,
the son we destroyed
not even there.

During the Empty Years

after Thomas Transtrommer

the soul was a shadow
under the liver's dark dome.
Naked, timid,
it breathed only
when it thought of you.

During the empty years
the intellect faltered,
courage took a rain check,
but the body
crossed the room to you.

Nothing mattered then,
not even the vague idea
of right or wrong.

The sky could rage.
The earth could take back
her blessing, but the soul,
the soul,
had a new tweed suit.

Jane Hirshfield

Some Thoughts on Poetry, Permeability, Wholeness, and Healing

The 18th- century German aphorist Novalis wrote, "Poetry heals the wounds inflicted by reason." More recently, a friend wrote, in the midst of a difficult time in her life, "The world demands that we actively heal it and ourselves every moment." These statements seem to me life-giving. Reading them, I feel awakened, alert, encouraged in some profound way. It seemed worth thinking about why that is, and how that connects to this conference's larger conversation.

At the center of both sentences is the word "heal," and at the etymological root of "healing" and "health" is the idea of wholeness. Whatever is healed is restored to wholeness. And one of the most essential forms of wholeness in human life is the inseparability and interconnection of all things and beings—of body and spirit, of self and other, of culture and self.

The wholeness of healing, in a life or in art, is not about raising barricades or preserving the status quo, not about clinging to old forms of being, saying, or understanding—a child whose immune system is overly protected and insufficiently challenged, is, we are learning, a child who is as likely to end up with asthma as a child unprotected from environmental insult. Nor does wholeness imply some artificial or simplistic unity, in its life inside the living body or in its life inside art. Any living creature or living art is joined with all other existence in complex, nuanced, and beautifully ungainly ways. Life also takes place within a continual process of breaking down and remaking. Our bones remodel, our brains remodel, our muscles, our spirits, our cultures, our art forms. Our grammars of being and conception continually remodel. Even illness remodels us, for some new fate.

Stresses strengthen (if we survive them). And they renew. This ceaseless changing is what underlies the Buddhist teaching of no fixed self. The wholeness of living creatures is made by their changing, their shifting, their interpenetration of one with another. Each perishing moment gives rise to another; the transient self is connected to other transient selves; reconstruction and deconstruction are always the case. We need only look around, or into a mirror, and our own provisionality and malleability are there with us, looking back, right alongside our sense of a unique, continuing self.

Both are available to be seen by eyes open to looking. There is not then, I don't think, an argument between wholeness and destabilization, in our physical embodiment, or in our art forms. Wholeness of being includes and is permeable to both.

This junction is one reason why poetry—and all the arts—can enter so deeply into what is called the art of healing: the arts dwell at the crossroads between what in us is body, what in us is emotion, and what in us is mind, and also at the crossroads between what is knowable and what is not, what is nameable and what is not, what is balanced and what is not, what is fixed—or fixable—and what is not. Poems and stories both console and, if they are good at all, also challenge. Fairy tales terrify as well as enthrall. Creative words' exhilaration and instruction is to raise questions as much as answers. This is how they enlarge us. To step into this kind of wholeness, under any conditions, is in itself restorative, is health. Healing, I would add, is not the same as "cure." A person cannot die "cured," but they can die healed.

The arts, then, are not frivolous extras—they are steps that raise us into the fullness of life. Everyone here must know, I am sure, the Greek myth of Orpheus and Eurydice. It is no accident that, if anything could have returned Eurydice to life, it would have been the maker of a transcendently beautiful music. And no accident that when music fails in its own self-belief, restoration falters.

When Novalis said, "Poetry heals the wounds inflicted by reason," he was speaking against the literalism that does reduce a person to only body or to only mind; against the literalism that creates a sense of the self as only ego, separate from others and in need of either desperate preservation or desperate breaking down; against a literalism that leaves out art and art's powers, true health and true health's powers. Novalis's words press back against reason's twin weaknesses: the fallacy of believing we are merely meat and the equal fallacy of intellectual or spiritual disembodiment.

Put another way: The rational mind, necessarily, divides. It is its task to examine part by part, to be both unimpassioned and partial. That is intellect's strength—intellect can run blind trials without weeping, knowing someone may die because of what they are being given, knowing someone may die because of what they are not being given. And we need these forms of dispassionate truth. But the images, words, metaphors, and sounds of poems live only by passion, and by compassion and empathy—these subjects also talked about by almost all of us who have spoken this week. Poems link us, by shared knowledge and shared feeling, to one another, and also to creatures, mountains, tools, insects, and stones. They knit broader, wilder existence and all our own interior experience into a whole: a world that is at the same time phenomena, intelligence, feeling, music, body, spirit. Whether by mirror neurons or some other mechanism we do not yet and may never be able to name, words, when they come into poems, acquire an invisible and undeniable and irresistible wing-span, one that lifts and lofts meaning beyond the literal and the narrow.

Meaning also matters.

When the holocaust survivor Victor Frankl said that meaning, the finding of larger meaning, was what allowed those in the camps to survive, it was the kinds of meaning found in poems and stories that he meant—meaning that connects us not only to every part of our selves and psyches but also to something beyond our own selves and psyches. This is one of the wisdoms held in the sentence written by my friend: "The world demands that we actively heal it and ourselves every moment." The statement is not solipsistic—it knows that there is no healing of the self without an equal healing of others, of the world. And this healing, the sentence knows, is not passive—it is an active demand. Sometimes we hear that request, sometimes we are too tired, too distracted, too filled with despair. But the demand is always there, and one of our jobs as human beings is to hear it, and answer.

And still, in the hardest situations, under the duress of approaching death or a child's illness or the infinite capacity for cruelty that lives in the human heart alongside our infinite capacity for compassion, there is often no answer, or no rational answer. What there is is the answer held in part by works of literature, the re-membering (literally, the rejoining of what has been divided into parts back into a larger whole) that is held in stories, prayers, songs, rituals, the ceremonies of inclusion that art creates and holds—even seemingly disjunctive, disruptive, or fragmenting art, when it is effective, as we could hear in the poems that Robert Hass read last night.

I remember, very often, a chapter from Primo Levi's *Survival in Auschwitz*. It tells of a day when he struggles to recall a canto from Dante's *Inferno*, so he can recite it to a fellow prisoner as they go to fetch soup. They do not share a language, and Levi struggles not only to recall the canto but to bring the terza rima's meanings, sounds, the nuances of each word-choice, into his own poor French. He comes to this passage:

> Think of your breed; for brutish ignorance
> You were not made; you were made men,
> To follow after knowledge and excellence.

And he then writes that, saying these lines, "For a moment I forget who I am and where I am." This of course is not a forgetting at all. It is remembering something that had seemed irremediably lost. In his own hell, imagined and lived, one poet remembers humanness. In the different, later, hell-realm of Auschwitz, that earlier poet's centuries-old language and music restore humanness to another, unforeseeably distant in time. And there is something else to remember as well: there is no way to arrive at those lines, at this story, except by walking into and through the gates of hell. Yet this is not a heroic act, not Orpheus's attempt at rescue—it is an unavoidable part of any human fate.

That is the other permeability I want to speak of here. We do not find freedom by bracing ourselves against the hardness of our own lives, or by any manipulation of definition. We find it by intimate embrace of pain, grief, sorrow, loss, fear. Poems allow us to draw close what, if we had a choice, we might push away. They give us a way to speak in hell, and to speak of hell, and to speak at the same time the names and shapes of beauty, freedom, grace. Primo Levi while conjuring Dante is not a prisoner, he is free. And that freedom is the seed bed of creativity, of compassion, of self in the sense of what Buddhism calls Big Self, rather than small.

Remember also: Levi conjures Dante because he is trying to teach the lines to another. We help one another. This is the work of literature as well. In our most private reading, we know that the poem we read speaks not only for us. Someone has been before and left us a message, a cache as essential as food and matches and shelter. Or, in writing a poem, we ourselves construct the cache, for self, for other, of alchemical language that enlarges, liberates, alters. And if alteration of the outer is impossible, alteration of the inner remains open: outer circumstance cannot keep us from either wholeness or freedom. In a person shackled, bound, gagged, the heart can still shift. Poems pass hand to hand, mouth to ear, heart to heart, and with them passes their secret inclusions of fear, despair, uncertainty, pain and their secret inclusions of song, bravery, buoyancy, connection. If you look closely enough at any good poem you will find in it all these things, the full 360 degrees of a human life. And you will find the permeable willingness to know, to feel. Good poems and good stories allow us to slip past the guard dogs of our own hearts and our own ideas—writing them, and reading them alike, we find our way into a world where whatever happens, we need not be lonely, we need not be prisoner. All existence is with us, its infinite forms and names, helping, sharing, and changing our fate.

Notes on Contributors

Elizabeth Ackerson attended The Healing Art of Writing conference at Dominican University of California in 2010.

Anne Anderson has three degrees in nursing and is a Certified Family Nurse Practitioner. She was an Adjunct Professor at Santa Clara University Graduate School of Counseling Psychology. Mrs. Anderson taught "Counseling the Elderly and Their Families" and "Living with Chronic and Life Threatening Illness." She has supervised counseling interns and was an examiner for the California Board of Behavioral Sciences oral examination of candidates for MFT licensure.

Rebecca Ashcraft is a nurse in Surgical Intensive Care at the Kansas City VA Medical Center. She lives with her incredible partner (Joan Marie) in a cool, old house where they've raised a beautiful daughter (Joan Abi) and several generations of happy kitties (names too numerous to mention). Rebecca campaigns tirelessly against the rumored extinction of parentheses.

Claire Badaracco, PhD, (Rutgers/UC Berkeley) is the author of *Prescribing Faith: Medicine, Media and Religion in American Culture* (2008) and "Nutrition and Branded Wellness," a chapter in *Spiritualities and Social Change* (2011), ed. of *Quoting God: How Media Shape Ideas about Religion* (2006), three other books and numerous academic articles in the field of mass media and communication. She is a Full Professor in the College of Communication at Marquette University, currently working on a book on "Equanimity and Technology: Mind-body Equations," about poetry and the impact of contemplating words and images on inner peace and mental balance.

Joan Baranow, PhD, is an Associate Professor of English at Dominican University of California. Her poetry has appeared in *The Paris Review*, *Western Humanities Review*, *The Antioch Review*, *The Western Journal of Medicine*, and other magazines. Her poetry has also appeared in *Women Write Their Bodies: Stories of Illness and Recovery*, issued in 2007 by Kent State University Press. Her book, *Living Apart*, was published by Plain View Press. With her husband, physician and poet David Watts, she produced the PBS documentary *Healing Words: Poetry & Medicine*, airing nationally in 2008–2011.

LeeAnn Bartolini, PhD, is a Clinical Psychologist and a Professor at Dominican University of California. She was introduced to poetry via a high school teacher's love of Dylan Thomas and her Aunt Sheila Ryan Green's love of reading, writing, and teaching poetry. She has been writing poetry since adolescence, but has only recently become a serious student of poetry. She is convinced of the healing aspect of writing and reading poetry and is interested in the intersection of poetry and psychotherapy.

Madeleine Biondolillo attended The Healing Art of Writing conference at Dominican University of California in 2010.

Fran A. Brahmi is a published poet and informationist. She was raised in Los Angeles, did her undergraduate work at UCLA, her graduate work (MA in English) at Butler University and at Indiana University (MLS) and earned her PhD in Information Science at age sixty-one from Indiana University . She spent eight years in France and Algeria at the Pasteur Institute (Library Director at Institut Pasteur d' Alger) where she conducted business in French. She currently resides in Indianapolis and directs a narrative medicine 4th year elective at Indiana University School of Medicine where she is the Statewide Lifelong Learning Competency Director.

Abby Caplin, MD, practices Mind-Body Medicine in San Francisco, Califonia, where she helps people with chronic illness find their direction, strength and power. She holds a master's degree in Integral Counseling Psychology and is a Diplomate of the College of Mind-Body Medicine. Dr. Caplin's stories and poems have been published in *Pulse: voices from the heart of medicine/The First Year*, *Tikkun Magazine*, and RitualWell.org. She hosts a blog for people with chronic illness who are "up in the middle of the night, or down in the middle of the day": http://permissiontoheal.word-press.org. She says, "'It Sometimes Happens' emerged from experiences and observations during my medical education. 'Morning at Esalen' describes my appreciation of this wonderful California retreat center."

Catharine Clark-Sayles is an internist practicing in Marin County. She rediscovered poetry at forty. Her first book of poems, *One Breath*, was drawn from medical training and practice (Tebot Bach, 2008). *Lifeboat*, her second book is due out in 2011. Her poems have been published in *Runes*, *The Bellevue Review*, *The Journal of Medical Humanities*, *The Journal of General Internal Medicine*, and *The Western Journal of Medicine*. Dr Clark-Sayles was included in the Sixteen Rivers anthology, *The Place That Inhabits You*. She regularly publishes in the annual *Marin Poetry Center Anthology* and *The Poetry Farmers' Almanac*.

Brian Cronwall teaches English at Kaua'i Community College in Hawai'i. His poems have appeared in numerous journals and anthologies in Hawai'i, Guam, the Mainland United States, Australia, Japan, United Kingdom, and France.

Jen Cross is a writing workshop facilitator living in the San Francisco Bay Area whose writing appears in many anthologies and print periodicals. A certified Amherst Writers and Artists workshop method facilitator with an MA in Transformative Language Arts (Goddard College), Jen has facilitated transformative writing workshops for survivors of sexual trauma and others since 2002. Jen has used writing as a critical part of her own healing process; she believes in the potential of open-hearted writing communities to transform individual lives and create wider social change. Visit her website at www.writingourselveswhole.org.

Therese Jung Doan is a perpetual student and lover of life, poetry, and yoga. She lost her husband of 20 years to lung cancer. Since then, she returned to school and obtained a PhD in Nursing. She is currently on faculty at San Francisco State University. Her biggest success is having three sons who truly love each other and their mother.

Sharon Dobie is Professor of Family Medicine, University of Washington (UW). She has an active clinical practice, teaches residents and medical students, supports service learning programs, and does research relevant to health disparities. Her interests include social justice, narrative medicine, and nurturing careers with the underserved. Her degrees are BA (Mary Washington University), MA, City Planning (University of California, Berkeley), and MD (University of California, San Francisco). For her work mentoring student run service learning projects, she received the 2010 UW Sterling Munro Public Service Teaching Award. She has two sons, lives, swims, sings, writes, teaches, and practices in Seattle.

Suzanne Edison was awarded two grants in 2008 to complete a chapbook of poems that reflect living with a child with a chronic illness. Her work has appeared in *Pearl*; *Snow Vigate* anthology; *Drash: Northwest Mosaic*, Vol. II & III; *Crab Creek Review*; *Blood and Thunder: Musings on the Art of Medicine*; *Ars Medica*; and *Face to Face: Women Writers on Faith, Mysticism and Awakening*, eds. Linda Hogan and Brenda Peterson. Some of her work can be read online at www.dermanities.com, www.literary-mama.com, and www.washingtonpoets.org/owas/.

Ann Emerson lives in La Honda, California. She attributes discovering her vocation as a poet to having been given a terminal prognosis several years ago. Ann resides with two cats among foggy redwoods in a faeryland cabin visited by deer, heron, coyote, and puma.

John Fox is a poet and Certified Poetry Therapist. He is adjunct associate professor at the California Institute of Integral Studies in San Francisco. He teaches at John F. Kennedy University in Berkeley, The Institute for Transpersonal Psychology in Palo Alto, and Holy Names University in Oakland. John is author of *Poetic Medicine: The Healing Art of Poem-making* and is featured in the PBS documentary *Healing Words: Poetry & Medicine*. He presents at medical schools and hospitals throughout the United States. John served as President of The National Association for Poetry Therapy from 2003–2005. John is President of The Institute for Poetic Medicine. Find out more about his work at www.poeticmedicine.org.

Jan Haag is a creative writing and journalism professor at Sacramento City College, where she developed a class called "Writing as a Healing Art." She worked as a reporter and copy editor for newspapers and United Press International, as well as serving as editor-in-chief for Sacramento magazine. She holds a master's degree in English and Journalism from California State University, Sacramento. A poet and prose writer, Jan is the author of a book of poetry, *Companion Spirit*, and has completed a young adult novel set in British Columbia. She is an Amherst Writers and Artists affiliate who leads writing workshops in Sacramento.

Jane Hirshfield's seventh poetry collection, *Come, Thief*, appears from Knopf in 2011. Other books include *After*, named a best book of 2006 by *The Washington Post*; *Given Sugar, Given Salt*, a finalist for the National Book Critics Circle Award; and a now-classic book of essays, *Nine Gates: Entering the Mind of Poetry*. Her honors include fellowships from the Guggenheim and Rockefeller foundations, the NEA, and The Academy of American Poets. Her work appears in *The New Yorker*, *The Atlantic*, *Poetry*, *Slate*, *The New Republic*, and five editions of *The Best American Poetry*.

Warren Lee Holleman, PhD is Associate Professor and Director of the Program on Faculty Health & Well-Being at the M. D. Anderson Cancer Center, Houston. Dr. Holleman has published articles in *JAMA, Lancet,* and other journals, served as co-editor of *Fundamentals of Clinical Practice: A Textbook on the Patient, Doctor, and Society,* and is author of *The Human Rights Movement: Western Values and Theological Perspectives.* He holds an AB in history from Harvard University, an MA and PhD in Religious Studies from Rice University, and an MA in Marriage and Family Therapy from the University of Houston-Clear Lake.

Carol Howard-Wooten has been a Marriage and Family Therapist since 1982 and a stroke survivor since 1985. Over 800 stroke survivors have participated in her small group program. Keeping Hope Alive is a nonprofit 501(c)(3) she founded in 2001 to expand the work of assisting survivors and their families in re-visioning their lives. The Healing Art of Writing is the first writing workshop she has attended though she has written for herself for years. Her poem "Group" was included in *Wounded Healers,* (1994). She received a MAT from Harvard and a MA in Psychology from JFK University. She has a private practice in Kentfield, California, where she works with individuals and couples.

Louis B. Jones is the author of the novels *Ordinary Money, Particles and Luck,* and *California's Over,* all three *The New York Times* Notable Books. His writing recently appeared in *Santa Monica Review* and *The Threepenny Review,* and in the 2009 Pushcart Prize collection. His newest novel is *Radiance,* published in 2011 by Counterpoint Press. With Lisa Alvarez, he directs the Writers Workshops of the Community of Writers at Squaw Valley.

Muriel Karr has published two books of poems, *Toward Dawn* (2002) and *Shape of Pear* (1996), both available from Bellowing Ark Press, and a chapbook *Membrane* (BGS Press, 1994). A graduate of Reed College and Indiana University, she has been both a Fulbright Scholar and a Woodrow Wilson Fellow, and formerly taught French and German at colleges in Indiana and Maine. Born in Lowell, Massachusetts, in 1945, she now lives in the San Francisco Bay Area with her husband, jazz pianist and songwriter Ron Karr.

Lisa Kerr is an assistant professor in the Writing Center at the Medical University of South Carolina, where she also teaches humanities courses in literature and writing. Her chapbook, *Read Between the Sheets*, was published by the South Carolina Poetry Initiative/Stepping Stone Press in 2010 and features a series of poems about love and loss, medicine and miracle, illness and healing.

Julia B. Levine's latest poetry collection, *Ditch-tender*, was published by the University of Tampa Press. Her awards include the University of Tampa prize for her second collection, *Ask*; the Anhinga Prize and a bronze medal from *Foreword* magazine for her first collection, *Practicing for Heaven*; The Discovery/The Nation award; the Pablo Neruda Prize in poetry; and multiple Pushcart Prize nominations. Her work has been anthologized in several collections, most recently in *The Places That Inhabit Us* and *The Autumn House Anthology of Contemporary American Poetry*. She lives and works in Davis, California.

Ashley Mann says, I live in Kansas City, Missouri, with my husband Chris, and I am in my last year of medical school planning to pursue a career in surgery. I take a lot of inspiration from the patients I see every day, and I think their stories are far better than any that I could tell—I owe them a great debt.

A nurse in practice for thirty-five years, twenty of them in primary health care, **Veneta Masson** was a founder, director and, for most of two decades, family nurse practitioner in a small, mom-and-pop clinic providing office and home care to an inner-city neighborhood in Washington, DC. Out of that rich and intense experience, she began to keep a journal and, eventually, to write poems and essays. Though no longer in practice, Veneta continues to explore healing art through reading, writing, teaching and making music. More of her work can be found at www.sagefemmepress.com.

Charlotte Melleno has practiced psychoanalytic psychotherapy in San Francisco since 1980. A student of Zen Buddhism and published poet, her themes concern family, direct experience, and the universality of loss. Four years ago, she was felled by lung disease and chronic pain and is lifted by humor, reading fiction, and her connection to friends and family. Writing poetry with others nourishes her, especially at Tassajara with her Jane Gang, a group of poets who love to study with Jane Hirshfield. Charlotte is currently writing a memoir about love, loss, and reconciliation.

Marilyn Morrissey is a mother and nurse who lives and works as a School Nurse in Boston. In November 2004, her husband of twenty-five years, a physician, was diagnosed with metastatic, inoperable pancreatic cancer. He died eighteen months later at home after an arduous attempt to extend his life by days, weeks and months. She is writing about their dual experience as active participants and critical observers of their cancer journey within the medical care system. But, mainly, she is writing about the necessity of Hope and what happened to their marriage during those eighteen months.

Meg Newman, MD, worked at SFGH, as a clinician, from 1984 until 2008. She joined the AIDS Division in 1994 as a clinician-educator, developed and directed many programs for patients and trainees and was sidelined prematurely due to spinal disease. Meg was a profoundly devoted and much beloved clinician, educator, and colleague. She began writing in the spring of 2010, is currently engaged in learning the craft of writing, and appreciates the transformative nature of self-expression through the written word. She lives happily in San Francisco with her partner, Sherry Boschert, and their ever-amusing ocicat, Alli.

Martina Nicholson is delighted to be an obstetrician. She says, I constantly feel tugged by the mystery and spectacular holiness of it. I feel that I am almost always living in a sort of Advent, waiting for Christmas. I believe that God comes into the life of a family through a baby—and I feel great joy each time I get to witness this miracle. I am really looking forward to the time when I get to be a grandmother. So this story poured out, whole, from that space in my work. I have had a hard time writing about patients, and their lives. It somehow seems that I shouldn't violate the privacy of their story, of our doctor-patient relationship. So I was interested to come to the writing retreat to try to learn a little more, and attempt to write about the themes in my work. I am a poet, but maybe I will someday begin to write stories.

Sarah Paris is a Swiss-American writer and author of the novel "Ahnenbeschwörung," published in Switzerland in 2000. She has also worked as a journalist and a screenwriter. Her current focus is on poetry, including haiku. She lives in San Francisco.

Terri Pauser Wolf, RN, BSN works as an oncology nurse in Northern California. She has cared for patients in pediatric oncology, adult chemotherapy and radiation oncology. She is a graduate student in the inaugural class of the Betty Irene Moore School of Nursing at University of California, Davis studying health care leadership and facilitates Writing as Healing workshops for patients, caregivers and staff.

Larry Ruth works as a consultant in natural resource and environmental policy. For many years he taught, conducted research and handled programmatic responsibilities at the University of California, Berkeley. Publications include articles of federal wildland fire policy, ecosystem management, forest policy in the Sierra Nevada, and adaptive management. He taught courses in environmental policy and natural resource law, policy and institutions. Research interests include energy policy and climate change, development and analysis of ecologically sensitive approaches to resource management, ecosystems services, wildland fire policy, and the effectiveness of administrative regulation.

Ruth Saxey-Reese (Ruth Salter) lives on the boundary between sagebrush and civilization near Boise, Idaho. When she's not wrangling turkeys or chasing goats, she teaches writing to adults at Boise State University and local non-profit organizations and to children at summer writing camps. Her work has been nominated twice for a Pushcart Prize and has appeared in several periodicals and anthologies.

Amanda Skelton lives in Sydney, Australia. She graduated with a medical degree from the University of Western Australia in 1983 but currently writes full-time. Her essays have appeared in *Hunger Mountain* and *Alimentum*. She was a resident at Varuna, the Writers' House, and a general contributor at Bread Loaf Writers' Conference in 2010. Membership of the FEAST Australia taskforce allows her to maintain her interest in better treatment options for eating disorders.

Jennifer Stevenson came to UCSF five years ago to become a nurse. It takes a year; it's not easy. So afterward, to relax a bit, she became an emergency room nurse. She developed many skills, one of which was to listen to the stories of patients' lives. Letting them know they were not alone was often more effective in moderating pain than prescribing medication. That said, Jennifer knows the powers of morphine are great; however, the power of connection lasts longer. Jennifer Stevenson is close to completing her master's degree in nursing at UCSF.

Through her early work as a women's health advocate, **Mary Stone** became interested in the roles patients are expected to play and not play in their own healing. She pondered questions of patient agency during a long career as a biomedical writer and eventually returned to graduate school to study medical rhetoric, exploring how language functions in the power dynamics between health care providers and patients. Mary has taught writing at Northern Arizona University, Arizona State University, and Glendale Community College and currently participates in several community poetry groups in the Phoenix area.

Terese Svoboda's sixth novel, *Bohemian Girl*, will be published September 2011. She has produced a body of work that includes five books of poetry, novels, a memoir, a book of translations, and poetry documentaries. Called "disturbing, edgy and provocative" by *Book Magazine*, her work has been chosen for the Writer's Choice column in the *New York Times Book Review* and garnered numerous awards. She has taught at Sarah Lawrence, Bennington, William and Mary, San Francisco State, and elsewhere. She was very happy to be in the company of such a wonderful group of caregivers!

Raised in Singapore and trained in journalism, **Suzanne Tay-Kelley** began writing as a staff reporter for the Los Angeles Times and the Oakland Tribune. Following postgraduate studies at UCLA/Anderson School of Management and UCSF, she dove into healthcare as a management/new ventures consultant with PricewaterhouseCoopers and Kaiser Permanente, then a cardiac and surgical oncology nurse at UCSF and the SF VA Medical Center. She is now a novice rheumatology nurse practitioner in private practice. She enjoys her patients, travel, photography, haiku, and tai chi, but mostly hanging with family.

Joanna Steinberg Varone is a writer, legal advocate, and social activist who practiced family law and mediation for several years before having to take disability due to the debilitating symptoms of multiple sclerosis. A graduate of Duke University (AB 1998) and Washington University School of Law (JD 2002), she is at work on her first book, a medical memoir-in-stories. She resides in Mount Olive, NJ with her husband, Jonathan, and can be contacted via e-mail at joanna.varone@alumni.duke.edu.

David Watts's second book of stories, *The Orange Wire Problem*, along with *Bedside Manners*, forms a body of work which explores the intricacies of the art of medicine. He has published four books of poetry and a CD of "word-jazz." He is an NPR commentator on *All Things Considered*, a producer of the PBS program *Healing Words: Poetry & Medicine*, a gastroenterologist at UCSF, and a classically trained musician. He has been an on-camera television host and a medical columnist for the *San Francisco Chronicle*. A volume of avant-guard poetry, *sleep not sleep*, was published under the pseudonym, Harvey Ellis, by Wolf Ridge Press. He lives in Mill Valley, California with his wife, Joan Baranow, and his two sons.

Wendy Patrice Williams, writer, public speaker, and workshop facilitator, has recently completed the manuscript of her medical memoir entitled *The Autobiography of a Sea Creature*. An accomplished poet, she has published two chapbooks, *Some New Forgetting* and *Bayley House Bard*. Her blog, Living in the Aftermath of Infant Surgery at http://myincision.wordpress.com, features inspiring words of healing highlighted with original artwork. She has been chosen to be an editor for the upcoming Fearless Books Poetry Series Volume Three, *Turning the Page: Poems of Trauma, Survival and Recovery*. She currently teaches English at the College of Alameda in California.

Lightning Source UK Ltd.
Milton Keynes UK
UKOW050800260712

196593UK00001B/28/P